Collins

need to know?

Sleep

Doctor Chris Idzikowski

Collins

First published in 2007 by Collins
an imprint of
HarperCollins Publishers
77–85 Fulham Palace Road
London w6 8jb

www.collins.co.uk

Collins is a registered trademark of HarperCollins
Publishers Ltd

09 08 07
4   3   2   1

A catalogue record for this book is available from
the British Library

Editor: Miren Lopategui
Designer: Jerry Goldie
Series design: Mark Thomson
Artwork: Ome Design

ISBN-10: 0-00-720223-7
ISBN-13: 978-0-007202-23-2

Printed and bound by Printing Express Ltd,
Hong Kong

Contents

Introduction

Sleep and wakefulness are two sides of the same coin and just about everyone has had a problem with them at one time or another. For many people the difficulties associated with sleep – sleeplessness, sleepiness, tiredness, fatigue – are short-lived and manageable while for others they become chronic and very hard to cope with.

People who need more than the average amount of sleep, say 9–10 hours a day tend to get little sympathy from those who get by on less. The latter, the 'short' sleepers, cannot understand why more is necessary to feel, function and look well. They are likely to know what it is like only when they cannot get enough sleep or their sleep is disrupted, such as from long commutes which do not leave much time for work and sleep, illness, jet lag, shift work, caring for others, etc. They have managed so they will wonder why it is not possible for others to cope – of course, they might lack insight because they are themselves chronically sleep-deprived; rather like someone who has drunk a little alcohol and thinks they are performing as well as before. Hence 'long' sleepers have a problem, as do 'average' sleepers if their sleep is disrupted and they are not getting enough. Those people with sleep disorders such as insomnia, narcolepsy, sleep apnoea (stopping breathing during sleep) or restless legs will be similarly aware that people who don't have these disorders seem not to care.

Well, this book does care and its aim is not only to help both the sufferers from sleep disorders but also those who want to feel better rested. After all, it has been shown that daytime napping improves mental performance later in the day. The book takes a systematic approach by first exploring what sleep is, its patterns and different stages. This enables readers to understand what their sleep problem is as well as enabling them to work out solutions for themselves. Chapter 2 runs through all those factors that impact on sleep. Sleep varies over our lifetimes and Chapter 3 examines these changes; it helps to understand whether there is a natural process at work or an underlying problem.

Chapter 4 starts to look at solutions that may not necessarily require medical aid or intervention. Chapter 5 delves even deeper and provides some self-assessment procedures that may give an idea of what is causing the sleep problems.

The field of sleep medicine has grown over the last decade or so. In the US it has become a medical speciality. In the UK, on the other hand, expertise runs across a number of specialities, ranging from general practice to respiratory medicine, ENT surgery, psychiatry, neurology and occupational medicine. Sleep medicine has developed in a way that is shared across countries and Chapters 6 and 7 deal with what are now considered sleep disorders and their specific solutions.

Disturbed or shortened sleep not only has an impact on mental performance, both in terms of concentration and increased risk of car accidents,for instance, but it is also associated with diabetes, obesity, heart disease and strokes. Problems with sleep should be tackled and this book shows how to go about this.

1 Knowing the basics

With our 21st-century lifestyles and the ever-increasing need to juggle work and family commitments, getting a good night's sleep has never seemed more important, yet although we spend a third of our lives asleep, research in this area is still relatively new. What really happens when we are asleep? And why is sleep so important? Although much of this fascinating and complex subject remains a mystery, scientists now have some of the answers to these all-important questions.

Understanding sleep

Sleep is essential for our survival and wellbeing. We all know it makes us feel good, alert and able to cope with our waking lives. But why is it so important? What are the benefits of sleep and what happens when we don't get enough?

must know

Animal sleep

- Sleep is so essential to animals that Nature has made special arrangements to enable it to happen. Horses' tendons are specially adapted to allow them to sleep standing up; similar adaptations allow South American sloths to sleep upside down, and migratory birds to sleep on the wing. Dolphin brains are so constructed to enable them to swim continuously while breathing (half their forebrain goes to sleep while the other half remains awake).
- The amount of sleep animals need varies according to their size. Elephants sleep for four hours, for instance; rats for 14.

Why sleep?

Sleep is not an optional extra. Like the food we eat and the air we breathe, it is a fundamental need. Sleep is essential for all living beings. Studies on animals have shown that sleep provides a period of enforced quietness in which they can hide from predators, and that sleep exists in all varieties of mammal, irrespective of their size, temperament and habitat.

The generally held view is that sleep energizes and revives, providing us with an enforced time of rest that allows us to recharge our batteries to cope with the everyday business of living. But many scientists argue that to think of sleep entirely in terms of rest is misleading, because it is also an active period when the restoration and repair of body tissue takes place. It is during sleep, for example, that growth hormones are released in developing babies and children.

There is also evidence to suggest that sleep plays a significant role in brain development, and that learning may improve after sleep. In experiments carried out in the UK and USA, subjects who were allowed to sleep after learning new information were found to have a better recall of the data they had learned than those who had not slept.

To most of us, the benefits of sleep are evident from the way we feel after a good night's rest. But perhaps a better way to understand the role of sleep is to look at what happens when we *don't* sleep.

Effects of sleep deprivation

Classic sleep deprivation experiments consist of depriving subjects of one night's sleep, then asking them to listen to about 1800 bleeps for an hour or so. About 40 of the bleeps are a second shorter than the others, and these are the ones the subjects have to react to. (Most errors of detection generally occur in the last 15 minutes of the task.) Experiments such as this have proved useful to scientists' understanding of the consequences of lack of sleep. Findings have shown the main short-term effects to be as follows:

- **General lack of wellbeing**. Lack of sleep can cause fatigue and grogginess.
- **Concentration and vigilance**. Experiments have invariably shown damaging effects in these areas. People who have been sleep-deprived are more likely to have difficulty taking in information and to make mistakes at work. In real-life situations requiring constant vigilance, such as driving, the dangers are obvious. Statistics show that 20 per cent of all road accidents are caused by fatigue and that many of these accidents will lead to fatalities.
- **Memory**. Many people complain that they are more forgetful when they do not get enough sleep. This could be down to a concentration problem but it may also be that sleep deprivation makes it more difficult to retrieve information from the brain's memory store.

must know
Rest and sleep
Scientists are baffled about the role of rest in sleep, as the amount of energy saved during sleep is only 100 kcal – the same number of calories as in a large piece of toast.

must know

Sleep deprivation
- 20-25 hours of sleep deprivation reduces mental performance to the same level as someone with a blood/alcohol concentration of 0.1 per cent, which is greater than the current maximum for legal driving in the UK – 0.08 per cent.
- The US Department of Transportation estimates that 100,000 accidents every year are caused by people feeling fatigued and/or drowsy, and that it leads to 4 per cent of all traffic-related deaths.

- **Mood.** Lack of sleep can lead to irritability and over-anxiety, which can have damaging effects on your social life, family and other relationships.
- **Immunity.** Evidence suggests that lack of sleep may affect the immune system. After vaccination, subjects who may have been sleep-deprived have 50 per cent fewer antibodies than those who have slept adequately. Sleep and the immune system are strongly linked; bacterial cell walls can stimulate the sleep centres directly.
- **Rational decision-making.** Studies show that sleep deprivation can affect general judgement and decision-making abilities, and that people who are sleep-deprived have difficulty in responding to rapidly changing situations. The real-life consequences can be grave. Fatigue is now known to have been a contributory factor in many international disasters such as the nuclear explosion at Chernobyl, the *Exxon Valdez* oil spill and the *Challenger* shuttle explosion.

Apart from these common short-term effects of sleep deprivation, there are also long-term consequences. American research suggests that long-term sleep deprivation (defined as interrupted sleep over a period of about a year) may be linked with obesity. Studies carried out at Colombia University have shown that 73 per cent of people who sleep only 2–4 hours a night are more likely to be obese than those who sleep for seven hours. The reason is unclear but it may be because chemicals that play a key role in appetite and weight gain are released during sleep. Other long-term consequences include extreme anxiety, depression, specific sleep-related disorders and even psychosis.

Key turning points in sleep research

Progress in sleep studies changed significantly when it was found that the brain's activity could be measured objectively. Here is a summary of the main findings that led to this discovery.

- In the 19th century, British researcher **Richard Caton** measured the brain's electrical activity by placing sensors on to the scalp's surface. He noted that the activity was not constant but increases and decreases over time.

- In the late 1920s, German psychiatrist **Hans Berger** measured brain activity in the belief that it would help him to calculate psychical energy. Largely discredited, he tragically committed suicide. However, his work on measuring the electrical activity of the brain was pivotal in the development of sleep research.

- In 1939, while working at Chicago University, **Nathaniel Kleitman** – often called 'the father of sleep' – published the first major book on sleep, *Sleep and Wakefulness* (1939). The generally held view of the scientific and medical establishment was that sleep is a passive condition. Kleitman was one of the few people in the world working on sleep at the time.

- In 1953, PhD student **Eugene Aserinsky**, while working with Kleitman, noted that the eyes move rapidly during sleep, eventually leading to the name of this state as Rapid Eye Movement (REM) sleep. Around this time, **William (Bill) Dement** joined them and all three were involved in the discovery that subjects awoken out of REM sleep often report dreaming – a turning point in knowing, as opposed to inferring, what goes on in the mind.

must know

REM and dreams

The discovery in the late 1950s/early 1960s of the connection between REM sleep (see page 20) and dreaming was one of the most exciting in sleep science because it proved without doubt that the brain was active during sleep. The findings marked the beginning of a new impetus in sleep research which lasted through the 1960s, when psychedelia was much in vogue. By the 1970s, interest had declined.

How sleep works

Sleep is a highly complicated but ordered process that is controlled by special wakefulness and sleep centres in the brain that work in tandem with hormones and our own internal body clock. The main players in this fascinating process are described below.

must know

24-hour cycle
Most living organisms, plants and animals, live according to a 24-hour cycle that is dominated by light and darkness. Even death can be part of this cycle, with cardiac arrests and strokes occurring mainly between 6 a.m. and 12 noon – perhaps because this is when blood tends to clot most.

Clocks, cycles and rhythms

We are all governed by a 24-hour cycle called a 'circadian rhythm', taken from the Latin words *circa*, meaning 'around', and *die*, meaning 'day'. Circadian rhythms underpin everything, from hormone production to when we feel like getting up or going to bed. Our body temperature has a 24-hour rhythm too; minimum body temperature usually occurs around 4 a.m., maximum body temperature around 10–11 p.m. Sleep also roughly follows a 24-hour rhythm.

For most of us, a typical cycle means falling asleep between around 11 p.m. and midnight, and waking up between 6 a.m. and 8 a.m., indicating that we are biologically programmed to be able to fall asleep and wake up at around those times. However, not all clocks keep the correct time, and the biological clock is no exception. It generally runs a little 'slow' but is kept to the right time relative to light and darkness by 'synchronizing' cues called 'zeitgebers'. Dawn light is one of the most important and well-understood cues that our body responds to, but the onset of darkness (which stimulates the production of melatonin from the pineal gland) also has a role to play. Other zeitgebers are exercise, meal-times, social interactions, sounds, and possibly changes in temperature. Sleep itself may be a weak zeitgeber.

Sleep and wakefulness

Working with the ebb and flow of the circadian rhythm are special sleep and wakefulness centres, which are located in a part of the brain called the hypothalamus. The sleep centre is in the same region of the brain that controls temperature (which may be why you sometimes can't sleep if you are too hot) and the wakefulness centre is near the part that is associated with activity. In an ideal world, the sleep centre will shut down during the day, when the wakefulness centre opens, and open at night, when the wakefulness centre closes. Not surprisingly, good sleepers have strong day-time wakefulness and night-time sleep systems. But if these centres have been damaged (through, say, over-use of caffeine, alcohol or drugs, or due to illness or age), you are likely to have sleeping problems.

The brain's sleep centres

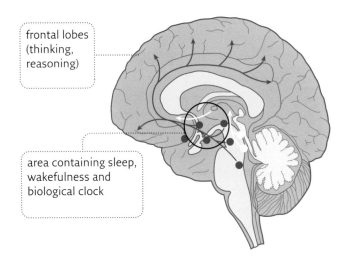

frontal lobes (thinking, reasoning)

area containing sleep, wakefulness and biological clock

The brain's metronome

The suprachiasmatic nucleus (SCN), is the brain's master biological clock, or metronome. It helps to synchronize sleep with the circadian rhythm, as well as regulating many of the bodily functions that affect sleep, such as hormonal secretion and body temperature. Made up of about 20,000 nerve cells, the SCN is located in the brain's hypothalamus, just behind the eyes, and is immensely important; if it is destroyed, 24-hour rhythms break down. It keeps time with daylight and is believed to work particularly closely with the wakefulness centre of the brain. Scientists also believe it 'instructs' the pineal gland to release melatonin, the hormone that signals the onset of darkness.

In 2002, a group of scientists discovered that the SCN is directly connected to a receptor in the retina sensitive to blue light (light from the sky), which enables the brain to identify whether it is light or dark. In blind people, who have damaged retinas, the SCN does not synchronize with daylight and so their ability to sleep is affected.

must know

Cues
The brain's metronome or clock runs slowly. Various cues such as light, exercise and food intake keep it synchronized with day and night.

The role of melatonin

Melatonin is secreted by the pineal gland in the brain (often known as the 'third eye' in reptiles because of its sensitivity to light), and is the hormone that 'tells' the brain it is dark. Secretion starts when it gets darker, peaks in the middle of the night and stops at dawn. Melatonin is believed to be an important synchronizer of other circadian rhythms and is closely connected with Seasonal Affective Disorder (SAD) and jet lag.

Seasonal Affective Disorder (SAD)

Seasonal affective disorder, or SAD, is a condition in which people suffer depression, insomnia and lethargy in the winter months – hence its alternative name, 'winter depression'. Normal circadian rhythms dictate that we get up in the light and go to bed in the dark. This is fine in the summer, but, in the case of SAD sufferers, the lack of light in winter is believed to disrupt their body clock so much that getting up on dark winter mornings proves impossible. The problem is believed to be caused by a disruption in their production levels of melatonin, the hormone which acts as the brain's and body's signal for darkness. Melatonin is normally produced at night, but in 80 per cent of SAD sufferers, melatonin levels peak just when it's time to get up. SAD is often treated with light therapy, in which sufferers are subjected to bright light. The light is believed to block the production of melatonin, which kick-starts and resets the body clock.

The role of serotonin

Serotonin as a precursor of melatonin is one of the brain's chemical messengers and has a major effect on the way the brain works, specifically affecting mood and sleep. (Other chemicals in this group include noradrenaline, dopamine and histamine.) It is produced in the brain from trytophan, an essential amino acid found in certain foods, and levels in the body are negatively affected by poor diet and stress. Lack of serotonin may lead not only to insomnia, but to anxiety and depression, which are in turn two of the greatest disruptors of sleep. Often known as the 'feel good' hormone, serotonin is Nature's own Prozac, and is a crucial in the way many of the more recent antidepressant drugs, known as Selective Serotonin Re-uptake Inhibitors (SSRIs), work.

did you know?

• Serotonin is one of the oldest brain chemicals around. Serotonin neurones existed in animals that appeared on earth 500 million years ago.
• Women produce up to a third less serotonin than men.

What happens when we sleep

Doctors and scientists can now record the activity of the brain in sleep by means of an electro-encephalogram or EEG. Using EEGs in this way has revolutionized our understanding of sleep.

The stages of sleep

In an electro-encephalogram (EEG), electrodes are glued to a person's scalp and then connected to powerful amplifiers that measure brain activity. Their output used to be printed on paper, but can now be seen on a computer monitor in the form of a graph called a hypnogram, or polysomnograph, which shows the brainwaves emitted during sleep. Eye activity and muscle tone are also recorded.

Using the EEG in this way has shown that people have two different kinds of sleep: non-REM (Rapid Eye Movement) sleep and REM, or dreaming, sleep, and that they go through five different stages within these two main types: Stage 1 (drowsiness), Stage 2 (light sleep), Stages 3 and 4 (deep sleep, sometimes called delta or slow-wave sleep) and Stage 5 (also known as REM sleep).

Stage 1: drowsiness

This is a short transitional stage, lasting only about 10–15 minutes. Your brainwaves will start to slow down from the normal 'alpha rhythm' measurement of 8–12 cycles per second, your muscles will start to relax and your eyes begin to roll. Polysomnographs taken at this stage show a 50 per cent reduction in activity compared to when awake. Although your eyes will be closed, if you are aroused from sleep at

must know

Deep sleep
- Deep sleep usually occurs during the first three hours and takes up to 20–25 per cent of the night.
- Stage 2, or light sleep, occupies around 50 per cent of the night.
- REM sleep occupies around 25 per cent of the night.

this stage you may feel as if you have not slept at all.

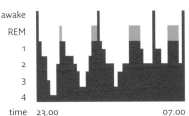
Hypnogram

Stage 2: light sleep

As you descend further into sleep, the relaxed alpha rhythm is replaced by a faster wave form of 12–14 cycles per second called a 'sleep spindle' (because of the spindle shape it makes on the computer screen). At this point the systems that maintain wakefulness are letting go and the sleep-promoting systems are switching on. This stage usually lasts 30–40 minutes.

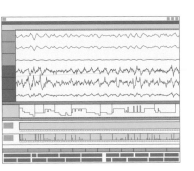
Set of traces

Stages 3 and 4: deep sleep, delta or slow-wave sleep

Slow-wave sleep lasts for roughly the first three hours of the night and it is very difficult to wake people up from it. People who are woken at this stage often act quite strangely, almost as if they are drunk.

At the deep-sleep stage, the EEG shows high-amplitude slow waves. The mind begins to drift, thoughts are unfocused, and the brain becomes 'dormant'. A person in this stage of sleep tends to stop moving and their postural muscles relax. Heart rate and breathing slows, the body temperature 'thermostat' in the hypothalamus is lowered and body temperature reduced. Kidney function decreases and less urine is produced.

must know

Ultradian rhythm
Scientists believe there may be a brain rhythm that is mainly revealed during sleep as a 90-minute REM cycle. As this lasts less than 24 hours it is known as an 'ultradian rhythm' (*Ultra* from the Latin for 'beyond'). Dreams occur on a roughly 90-minute cycle.

Stage 5: Rapid Eye Movement (REM) sleep

Stage 5 sleep is commonly known as Rapid Eye Movement, or REM sleep, named after the darting eye movements that have been observed in people in this sleep stage. It appears after 80–90 minutes' sleep in recurring phases known as an REM cycle. It initially lasts for about ten minutes, then increases in length, with the final one lasting for about an hour. In young adults, REM sleep can last for up to two hours in total.

For many sleep scientists, REM sleep is the most interesting and exciting of all sleep stages, for this is when dreaming occurs, and is when the brain is most active. In fact, curiously, EEGs taken at this time are more similar to those taken during wakefulness than at other sleep stages. The brain shows increased cerebral metabolism, cerebral blood flow, intracranial pressure and brain temperature, and many parts of the brain that control functions such as heart rate, blood pressure, breathing, body and brain temperature and sweating are less well regulated than at other times. Even sexual organs are aroused and men often have penile erections. In fact, there was a time when REM EEGs were used to determine whether men's impotence was physical or psychological, though this has all changed in recent years with the introduction of Viagra.

REM sleep and dreaming

Scientists believe we dream during REM sleep, and that the dreams become more vivid as the sleep stage progresses. Most REM sleep occurs towards the end of the night and can sometimes reach its peak in the early morning, (which is why you can often remember dreams clearly just as you wake up). But the memory of the dream usually fades within minutes.

must know

Are you a dreamer?
If you don't think you dream, try setting your alarm clock at 15-20 minutes earlier than your usual morning wake-up time. This will almost certainly ensure that you will be awoken out of REM sleep. Go to bed preparing yourself to remember what is in your mind when you wake up. When the alarm goes off, think about what has been going through your mind.

Sigmund Freud and dreams

Although he originally trained as a doctor, Sigmund Freud (1856–1939) is best known for his study of the mind, and is often referred to as the father of psychoanalysis. Freud believed that the mind consisted of three main elements: the ego (the conscious self), the superego (the mind's moral guardian) and the id (psychic and unconscious mental energy), and that the demands of the id, left unchecked during sleep, were expressed in dreams.

In Freud's psychodynamic theory, dreams symbolized unconscious thoughts and mental processes, and interpreting their meaning was a 'royal road' to understanding the subconscious mind. One of Freud's contemporaries, Carl Jung (1865–1961), formulated the idea of the 'collective unconscious' (a reservoir of memories and experiences), his list of the many recurring themes in dreams including: water, being trapped, travelling, running, being chased, death, choking, falling, houses, flying, nudity, being late and sex.

Freud's influence on psychiatric thought has now largely declined, but his book *The Interpretation of Dreams* (1900) remains one of the most significant works of the 20th century.

REM sleep has often been described as paradoxical because it has many contradictions. Although EEG readings show that the brain is so active at this time that it may be using even more energy than during wakefulness, the muscles, by contrast, are completely paralyzed, apart from rapid eye movements and the odd, involuntary twitching of fingers. Since vivid dreams also occur at this time, some people believe the muscle paralysis is there to stop the dreams from being physically acted out.

did you know?
During REM sleep your brain is as active as when you are awake.

Dreaming through the ages

Dreaming has intrigued and fascinated people for thousands of years before the works of Sigmund Freud, and many of the world's greatest civilizations and religions have used dreams to guide their everyday lives. Let us look at some of the most famous examples below.

did you know?

An ancient Hindu tale that is still relevant today describes three states of mind: the state of wakefulness (*vaiswanara*), when a person perceives 'what is presented to them by their senses', the state of dreaming sleep (*taijasa*) 'which can reflect in the mind what has happened in a person's past', and the state of dreamless sleep (*prajna*) when 'the veil of unconsciousness envelops thought and knowledge, and the subtle impressions of the mind apparently vanish'.

The ancient Egyptians

By around 2000 BC, the ancient Egyptians were already transcribing their dreams on to papyrus. Egyptians believed that dreams brought messages from the gods and that dreaming was the best way of attaining divine revelation. They developed methods for inducing or incubating dreams, including building sanctuaries that had special beds for dreaming.

The ancient Greeks

Sanctuaries and shrines for promoting dreams were also adopted by the Greeks, who in addition had specific dream rituals. Those entering the Shrine of Apollo at Delphi were required to abstain from sex, or eating meat, fish and fowl two days before. Once in the shrine, they made an animal sacrifice to the god from whom they wanted to receive the dream and would then sleep on the skin of the sacrificed animal, sometimes near the statue of the appropriate deity. The Greek god Hypnos was thought to bring sleep to mortals and his son Morpheus was said to send warnings and prophecies to those sleeping in the temples.

The early Christians

The Judeo-Christian tradition also used dreams as a guide to waking behaviour, most notably in the story of Jacob's dream of the ladder going up to heaven recounted in Genesis, which was seen as a turning point in his spiritual development. Various books from the Old Testament used dreams for guidance – it was assumed that the conventional way for God to communicate with his people was through dreams. Dreams were similarly used in the New Testament; for example, in stories of the Flight into Egypt and the dream of the Magi at the birth of Christ.

In the first century AD, Ignatius of Antioch dreamt of angels singing alternating chants and introduced this antiphonal singing in monastic communities as a consequence. (Ignatius could possibly be described as one of the early sleep researchers as he claimed that all people dreamt and that this could be observed by their movements when asleep!) And in the fourth century, Chrysostom declared that dreams were symbolic reflections of a spiritual world.

The early philosophers

The early philosophers had opposing views on dreams. Plato argued that there was a world beyond the physical one and that it was possible to communicate with it through dreams, while Aristotle argued that knowledge was gained through sense and reason and that there were no divine communication pathways of communication – dreams were just the remnants of an overly stimulating wakefulness. The debate still continues...

want to know more?

Take it to the next level...
- Chronotherapy 180
- Circadian rhythm disorders 139
- Light 38
- Light therapy 178
- Melatonin supplements 178
- Seasonal Affective Disorder (SAD) 17
- The work of sleep clinics 168

Other sources
- For professional sleep research societies, visit www.wfsrs.org
- To read specialist journals on sleep, visit www.journalsleep.org
- For brain basics and disorders, go to www.ninds.nih.gov or www.websciences.org/sltbr/
- For contemporary discussion and links on sleep, visit www.neuronic.com or read sleep blogs: scienceblogs.com/clock/

2 Why can't we sleep?

Surveys show that 95 per cent of us will suffer from sleeping problems at some point in our lives, and insomnia is cited as one of the main reasons for visits to the doctor. But what is insomnia? And, more importantly, why do we get it? All too often the answer lies within. This chapter looks at the important roles that Nature, lifestyle and environment have to play.

All about insomnia

Studies show that 50 per cent of us have symptoms of insomnia at any given time. We often use the word 'insomnia' when we miss one night's sleep. But what does insomnia really mean?

What is insomnia?

In normal usage 'insomnia' just means not being able to sleep. The inability to sleep can be caused by literally anything. Sometimes people talk about insomnia when they have not given themselves enough time to sleep, but when considered by a sleep disorder specialist, insomnia is often just regarded as a symptom and a cause is sought, e.g. depression (see page 156). Nowadays a sleep disorder specialist may regard insomnia as a disorder in its own right with very specific sleep-related causes (see pages 127–31). The changes in the usage of the word can cause confusion (particularly when surveys are conducted). An outdated classification simply described three types:

- **Transient insomnia** – short-term sleeping problems (usually lasting only a few days). Often caused by one-off changes in your sleep cycle, such as long-distance travel and jet lag, or illness. This is by far the most common type, and accounts for about 75 per cent of all cases of insomnia.
- **Short-term insomnia** – sleeping problems caused by a more prolonged period of stress, due to, say, financial problems or marital break-up. This can last for weeks.
- **Chronic insomnia** – the often inevitable result of untreated short-term insomnia. It can last for months, and, in rare cases, years. It is a long-term problem that often recurs.

did you know?
- Insomnia is the most common mental health problem in the UK.
- One in ten people will suffer from chronic insomnia at some point in their lives.

Sleeplessness and insomnia

It may be better to use two words: 'sleeplessness' for the times that sleep is impossible, but you know why; and 'insomnia' for the times that you do not know why you cannot sleep. Some reasons for sleeplessness include:

- lifestyle (work, shifts, caring for an invalid, children)
- poor sleeping environment (noise, uncomfortable mattress, etc.)
- stress (bereavement, divorce, etc.)
- a poor diet
- stimulants, medicines and drugs

As a general rule, a good way to find out if you have true insomnia is to ask yourself if there is any obvious reason for your sleeping problems. If not, and you have had the problem for a few weeks, then you are likely to be suffering from the condition.

Diagnosing insomnia

Insomnia can develop from sleeplessness, and often patients will know when their sleep problems started but cannot understand why they have not gone away. Psychiatrists rarely diagnose insomnia but when they do the following conditions must be met:

- The time it takes to get to sleep must be more than 30 minutes. Total sleep time during the night is usually between three to six hours. The sleep may be unrefreshing.
- The problem must occur three or more nights a week.
- The insomnia causes major problems in daytime functioning (socially, at home, at work).
- It must have lasted for three months or longer.
- There are no environmental, lifestyle, medical or psychiatric causes for the problem.

must know

Using sleeping pills
Prescription of sleeping pills costs the UK about £22.4 million per year. About 15.5 million prescriptions are written. Taking sleeping pills has been shown to increase the risk of road accidents (last year there were 32,220 serious injuries and deaths on UK roads).

The role of Nature

Understanding when our bodies are working against us can sometimes be half the battle when trying to understand why we can't sleep. Here are some of the natural factors that can affect sleep.

must know

Women and sleeping
Polls carried out in the USA by the National Sleep Foundation found the following:
• Almost three out of four women get less than eight hours' sleep a night.
• Sleep is disturbed for 2.5 days on average during the menstrual cycle.
• More women complain of sleep problems during menstruation (71 per cent) than during the week preceding menstruation (43 per cent).
• Sleep-disrupting conditions such as anxiety and depression are twice as likely to occur in women than in men.

Gender

It is a sad fact of life that you are more likely to have sleep problems if you are a woman. The reason for this is partly due to the female bodily cycles. Much of women's lives is governed by the sex hormones oestrogen and progesterone, and hormonal fluctuations, as in the menstrual cycle, pregnancy and the menopause, can severely affect sleep either directly, or through their effects on anxiety and general mood. Pre-menstrual women commonly report sleeping difficulties in the week before their period starts, but even women who don't suffer from pre-menstrual symptoms can still take longer to fall asleep, wake more often and feel less refreshed after sleep during the second phase of their cycles. Sleep disturbances also become more common during the menopause, when women report waking up more often at night and feeling more tired during the day.

Studies on the effects on sleep of Hormone Replacement Therapy (HRT) and oral contraceptives have shown that these hormones have direct effects on the brain. Oestrogen has widespread effects on mental performance, mood, movement co-ordination and pain. However, the monthly fluctuation of oestrogen and progesterone impacts

on cognitive function, mood, appetite and temperature, as well as the sexual organs and breasts,
making it more difficult to work out how they affect
sleep directly.

There is evidence to suggest that women's role in
society may affect their sleep even more than
hormonal changes. The added pressures many
women face of juggling stressful jobs with their roles
as mothers and wives can often pose an intolerable
burden, exacerbated by the fact that many women
ignore their fatigue.

Age
Ageing can greatly affect sleep, with the number of
hours declining as you get older. While a young adult
will sleep on average for 7–8 hours, by old age this
will go down to about six. Quality of sleep is affected
too. Stage 4 sleep is reduced, and the proportion of
REM sleep, which makes up abut 50 per cent of baby
sleep, will, in the latter stages of life, go down to
15–20 per cent. Although the cause may be
inevitable, there are still steps you can take to
improve the situation (see Chapter 4).

General constitution
Your sleep is more likely to be poor if your general
health is poor, even if you are not suffering from a
specifically sleep-related disorder (see Chapter 6).
Conditions such as heart disease, general breathing
problems and arthritis can make it difficult to get
comfortable at night, and will almost certainly have
an impact on your sleep. Consult your doctor if this
becomes an issue. For many people emotional issues and
character make-up may come into play.

must know
Adult sleep
A recent US National
Sleep Foundation survey
looking at the relation-
ship of sleep problems in
adults aged between
55–84 found:
● Nearly one in four
adults had at least four
medical conditions.
● Depression, heart
disease, pain and
memory problems were
most associated with
insomnia.
● Ninety per cent of
those that did not have
any medical condition
thought their sleep
quality was good or
excellent. This went
down to 78 per cent if
they had 1–3 medical
conditions, and 59 per
cent if they had four or
more conditions.
● Obesity, arthritis,
diabetes, lung disease,
stroke and osteoporosis
were more likely to be
associated with other
sleep problems (e.g.
snoring, restless legs).

The role of diet

The role of food and drink in sleep is often overlooked but there is increasing evidence that healthy eating habits can have many beneficial effects. The first stage is to identify and eliminate the main sleep spoilers.

must know

UK safe limits for alcohol
• Men should drink no more than 21 units of alcohol per week (and no more than four units in any one day).
• Women should drink no more than 14 units of alcohol per week (and no more than three units in any one day).
• Pregnant women: if you have one or two drinks of alcohol (one or two units), once or twice a week, it is unlikely to harm your unborn baby. However, the exact safe limit is not known.

Alcohol

Drinking small amounts of alcohol (especially a glass of wine with meals) can be pleasurable, and its benefits well recognized. The problem comes when alcohol is drunk in large doses.

Drinking alcohol at night is commonly believed to be helpful for sleep. This is a myth. Drinking large doses may make you fall into a deep sleep straight away, but as soon as the immediate effects of the alcohol wear off (usually after 3–5 hours), you will wake up feeling exhausted, and your sleep is likely to be disrupted for the rest of the night. Drinking large amounts of alcohol can depress brain activity and induce unconsciousness. Breathing is also invariably impaired, leading to snoring. Alcohol also has a diuretic affect, which means that, depending on how much you've drunk, you could end up getting up to go the toilet several times during the night.

Caffeine

Caffeine is a very powerful stimulant that is known to cause the delay of sleep onset. Studies have shown that a dose equivalent to one cup of coffee taken at bedtime can both increase the time taken to fall asleep and decrease sleep quality, especially in non-REM deep sleep (see page 19). In a few individuals, a

How much alcohol is in your drink?

Sample drink	Quantity	Alcohol by volume	Units
Can of lager	500ml	4.00%	2
Glass of cider	500ml	4.00%	2
Alcopop	400ml	5.00%	2
X-Strong lager	500ml	8.00%	4
Glass of wine	160ml	12.50%	2
Cocktail	125ml	40.00%	5
Shot of spirits	25ml	40.00%	1

Note: A unit is 10ml of alcohol, whether it is spirits, lager or wine.

dose of coffee in the morning can also have an effect the following night, indicating that extremely low concentrations of caffeine can affect sleep. Like all stimulants, caffeine may make you feel increasingly alert during the day, but, as well as causing insomnia, prolonged, high-dose usage (more than six cups of coffee a day) can lead to the following nasty side-effects:

- persistent anxiety
- an inability to concentrate
- increased muscle tension
- diuresis (increased urination)
- agitation, excitement and panic attacks (with high doses)
- vertigo, dizziness, tinnitus, convulsions
- increased body temperature
- confusion, disorientation, paranoia
- palpitations
- nausea

watch out!

A good night's sleep does not result from high doses of alcohol. A night's sleep deprivation will enhance the effects of alcohol and after five nights of partial sleep loss, three drinks will have the same effect on your body as six would on a regular night.

Caffeine enters the bloodstream very quickly and can take between three and seven hours to leave the body. Its effects on people can be variable – some people regularly drink caffeine-laden drinks at night-time with no ill-effects; others cannot even drink one cup in the morning without it affecting them at night. Scientists believe this may be because caffeine-sensitive individuals metabolize the substance more slowly (see opposite, for factors involved in metabolizing caffeine).

Research shows that if you are not a habitual coffee drinker, the effects will be greater; and that caffeine metabolism varies with age (children, for example, tend to metabolize it more quickly).

Although caffeine is normally associated with coffee, it is found in medicines and many other foods and drinks, namely:

- tea
- chocolate, cocoa and all other chocolate-flavoured products
- over-the-counter stimulants (e.g. Pro-plus)
- painkillers (e.g. Anadin)
- herbal preparations (e.g. Guarin)
- some cola drinks
- Lucozade
- 'energy' drinks (e.g. Red Bull)

To find out how much caffeine you are really consuming, see the main caffeine offenders, opposite.

must know

Caffeine
- Caffeine is readily absorbed and peak concentrations occur 30–60 minutes in young adults after ingesting it. High doses slow the metabolism down and can remain in the brain for 9–15 hours.
- Percolated coffee usually contains more caffeine than instant. If the coffee grounds are boiled during preparation, as is common in Scandinavian countries, the caffeine content can be as high as 500mg per cup.
- Tea brewed directly from crushed leaves has more caffeine than tea produced with a tea bag.
- Plain chocolate contains more caffeine than milk chocolate.

The absorption and metabolism of caffeine

Varied or little effect

Heredity Caffeine metabolism is controlled by many genes and racial differences exist

Gender Exercise and stress have no reliable effect on the absorption or metabolism of caffeine

Pregnancy There are no placental barriers to caffeine so the foetus is continuously exposed

Slowers-down

Oral contraceptives, late pregnancy and liver disease cause caffeine to be eliminated more slowly

It has been thought that grapefruit juice, though not other citrus juices, slows down metabolism. The data for this has now proved controversial

Some drugs like cimetidine, disulfiram, even alcohol, may slow down caffeine metabolism

Speeders-up

Smoking induces liver enzymes which break caffeine down

Rifamprin

The main caffeine offenders

Foodstuff	Plant	Plant caffeine content w/w	Caffeine dose/ 'cup'
Tea	Dried leaves	1–5%	10–100mg (average 40mg)
Coffee	Beans	0.75–2.0%	30–150mg
'Decaffeinated' coffee	Beans	0.75–2.0%	5mg
Cocoa	Seeds	0.013–1.7%	2–50mg (average 5mg)
Chocolate	Seeds		2–63mg/50g
Cola drinks	Nuts	1.5–2.0%	25–100mg (synthetic)

did you know?

Coffee is an ancient commodity. In AD 575, about 500 years before it became a hot beverage, the crushed beans were mixed with fat and used by Ethiopian mountain warriors to provide an energy boost during long treks and warfare.

Sugar

Sugar can have a negative impact on sleep patterns because of its effect on insulin and blood sugar levels. It is released into the bloodstream to give you that instant 'high', but then departs from your system just as quickly, leaving you exhausted. In fact, you feel so tired that your instant impulse is to have yet another sugar fix to make you feel better. And so the cycle goes on. The continuing effect of these highs and lows can leave you feeling drained, or – depending on when you last had your sugar dose – over-excited, with pounding palpitations that stop you from sleeping. The disruptive impact on blood sugar levels can also cause sleep-disrupting hormonal imbalances in women. Sugar is found not only in biscuits and sweets, but also in fizzy drinks, refined wheat, tomato ketchup, baked beans and many processed foods. Read all food labels carefully.

'Good sleep' foods

There is some evidence to suggest that eating slow-release energy foods, or low glycaemic index foods, (foods that keep blood sugar levels stable), may improve general health and sleep quality (as well as helping the individual to lose fat). The idea is that the lower the glycaemic rating of a particular food, the more slowly energy, in the form of glucose, will be released into the body (see Low glycaemic index foods, opposite). Thus glucose and insulin levels are prevented from plummeting during the night, which may be beneficial for sleep. Foods such as turkey and dairy products may also be helpful, as they are high in tryptophan – the amino acid that the body uses to produce the sleep-inducing hormones serotonin and melatonin (see pages 16–17).

must know

Sugar

Sugar does not give you energy. A study carried out at Loughborough University, UK evaluated the energy-giving effects of sugar on ten healthy young adults. Their sleep was restricted to five hours the night before so that they would be sleepy in the afternoon, and half were given a 'high-energy' drink containing high levels of sugar but low levels of caffeine, and the other half a drink containing low levels of both. When submitted to vigilence and sleepiness tests the high-sugar drinkers made twice as many errors and showed higher levels of sleepiness than the control group, as well as delayed reaction times.

Low glycaemic index foods

Food	Carb (g)	Fibre (g)	Cal (kcal)
Granary bread, 1 slice	14	1.9	71
Rye bread, 1 slice	13.7	1.7	66
Chickpeas, small can, 200g	32.2	-	230
High-fibre bran, 40g	18.4	10.8	112
Rolled oats, 100g	62	7	368
Porridge (cooked and made with water) 100g	8.1	0.8	46
Apple, 1 medium	21	3.8	82
Avocado, half medium	8	3.4	160
Ham, honey-roast, 50g	1.4	0.5	68
Pumpkin seeds, 25g	11.8	1.1	143
Spaghetti, cooked weight 100g	22.2	-	113

What to eat when

When we eat can be as important as what we eat. This is a question of balance. Hunger can keep you awake, so having a light snack before you go to bed can be advisable. On the other hand, going to bed with a stomach that is over-full may cause indigestion and feelings of discomfort that will keep you awake all night, especially if you have eaten fatty and rich foods that make your digestive system work harder.

As a rule it is best to eat your main meal at lunch time or early evening, and to eat small amounts of light food at night-time. Snacking if you wake during the night is not a good idea. Your body may come to expect food at this time, and you will carry on waking up in the night to satisfy your hunger.

must know
Diet
Studies on the effect of milky or malted drinks on sleep appeared to show benefits. However, evidence does suggest that non-milky herbal teas are just as effective in promoting a good night's sleep.

Lifestyle

The way we live can provide a crucial pointer to our sleep problems. Stress, shift work, smoking and jet lag can all be contributing factors. It can be hard to change the habits of a lifetime, but when it comes to sleep, small changes can go a long way.

must know

Sleep in ex-smokers
Sleep disturbances and related daytime symptoms may leave the ex-smoker less able to cope with everyday stress, therefore increasing the likelihood of relapse. Studies have found that ex-smokers complaining of broken sleep are the most vulnerable.

Stress

This is by far the most common cause of insomnia, and can be short-term (caused, say, by the arrival of a new baby) or prolonged (juggling a career and family, or caring for someone who is ill).

Stress has been with us since ancient times, when our forebears used the natural 'fight or flight' response to deal with threatening situations such as attack. The causes of stress may be different now but the basic response is still there. 'Fight or flight' increases breathing rate, heart beat, and the production of the stress hormones cortisol and adrenaline; mental awareness is heightened and blood rushes to the muscles; the body is on red alert to deal with whatever crisis it is faced with. Doctors acknowledge that we all need some degree of fight or flight in our lives because it satisfies a primitive urge for survival. But prolonged stress can have damaging effects on both health and sleep. It is well documented that long-term stress can lead to anxiety and depression – two major sleep disruptors that can be the cause of many sleep-related disorders (see Chapter 6). Acknowledging when things have got out of hand and taking stress-relieving measures is the only solution (see Chapter 5).

Smoking

Despite the well-known risks of smoking, this still remains a major problem – mostly due to the highly addictive nature of nicotine itself, which can make it extremely difficult for habitual smokers to stop. Withdrawal symptoms can begin quickly – often within a few hours of the last cigarette – leading to sleep disturbances. The brain's nicotine receptors respond very rapidly to the lack of nicotine, which is why for habitual smokers the first cigarette of the day can bring the most relief, even though smoking in the night can cause disrupted sleep.

The combined impact of the brain's response to the lack of nicotine and the breathing problems that all smokers invariably suffer from mean that nicotine is most definitely not good for sleep.

Sadly, smoking is a vicious cycle that creates numerous problems. Many people start the habit because they find it useful for maintaining or increasing their alertness. (When inhaled, nicotine quickly stimulates the heart, brain and adrenal glands.) This is particularly true among young people and sufferers of sleep-related disorders. The need to boost alertness with nicotine reinforces the use of tobacco. Tobacco disturbs sleep, reducing daytime alertness, which in turn reinforces the use of tobacco. Apart from keeping you awake, there is evidence to suggest that nicotine may affect sleep in other, more indirect ways too. Smoking is believed to affect blood sugar levels, which can make you irritable, and smokers are also statistically more likely to be coffee-drinkers, the combined effect of nicotine and caffeine having a disastrous long-term impact on sleep duration and quality.

must know
NRT
Nicotine replacement therapy (NRT), which reduces the urge to smoke, is recognized as an effective aid to stop smoking, and increases cessation rates. Unfortunately, nicotine patches can sometimes be over-stimulating, leading to insomnia. The 24-hour patches are less problematic than the 16-hour ones, however.

Environment

Studies have shown that the sleeping environment can have a great impact on sleeping patterns. The degree of noise, vibration, light, humidity, or sharing a room with a partner who snores – all can have a significant part to play.

must know

Light and the retina

The retina consists of receptors that are sensitive to light. One group known as the ganglion cells are particularly sensitive to light, and in particular to blue light (such as that of the sky). These cells make a direct connection to the biological clock (see page 14) which controls the time that we are likely to sleep. About 20 per cent of light gets through the eyelids when the eyes are shut, which means that we can be affected by light and the time that we sleep even when we are in bed with our eyes shut!

Light

Light can have a profound effect upon our wellbeing, both consciously and unconsciously. The conscious effects of light have been known for many years. Numerous studies have shown that subjects exposed to bright light experience significant improvements in mood and a decrease in feelings of tiredness. Indeed, conditions such as Seasonal Affective Disorder (SAD – see page 17) are even treated by exposure to bright light. In recent years, scientists have learned that it is blue light (or natural skylight) that has the greatest effect on our sleeping patterns, because of the unique and very special influence it has on our internal bodyclock – the mechanism that determines what time we go to sleep at night and get up in the morning. (See The brain's metronome, see page 16).

Any disruption to the bodyclock can lead us believe that it is daytime rather than night, and to react accordingly. Blue light, it is believed, also inhibits the night-time secretion of melatonin, the hormone that signals the onset of darkness (see page 16), thus preventing or disrupting sleep. (When it is dark, melatonin secretion rises and peaks at the darkest time and then goes down until dawn, when the biological clock is reset to wake.) The effects of blue light are unconscious.

There are also conscious effects of perceived light: the brighter the light in your bedroom, the more alert and less sleepy you will feel. Taking lux as a measurement of light intensity (see the table below), normal indoor lighting measures around 200 'lux', while a cloudy day is around 10,000 'lux' – significantly lighter, which makes it crucial to block it out as much as possible when you go to sleep. If you cannot control the amount of light you are exposed to and don't want to hide your eyes with a pillow, consider using an eye mask.

In recent years, street and industrial lighting has increased dramatically, which has had a great impact on normal daylight hours and in some people can have the effect of disturbing the timing of their internal clocks. Again, an eye mask, thick curtains, or curtains with extra lining may help.

did you know?

Blind or visually impaired people have no internal bodyclocks because their retinas are so damaged that light cannot enter the brain. They will therefore have no natural sense of when to get up and when to go to bed.

The relative intensity of different forms of light

Illuminance	Example
0.00005 lux	Starlight
1 lux	Moonlight
400 lux	A brightly lit office
400 lux	Sunrise or sunset on a clear day.
1000 lux	Typical TV studio lighting
32,000 lux	Sunlight on an average day (min.)
100,000 lux	Sunlight on an average day (max.)

Note: Lux is a measure of the intensity of light.

There is some evidence to suggest that using coloured lighting may affect the 'colour temperature' of a room. Colours can be pleasing to some people and irritating for others so it is important not to be too assertive as to which are best. However, in general the warmer colours of sunset tend to be associated with deep sleep while the cooler colours of dawn are associated with darkness.

Humidity

One of the most common breathing-related sleeping disorders is asthma, which is often caused by allergens found in the faeces of house dust mites. The relative humidity of your surroundings will be the key factor that influences the prevalence of these mites, which can live in conditions where there is no liquid to drink as they can extract sufficient water from the environment if the humidity is high enough. Surveys in temperate climates show that mite prevalence varies according to seasonal fluctuations in indoor humidity. Mites are absent or rare in homes in dry climates unless use of evaporative coolers adds the moisture to the air that is necessary for their survival. Maintaining average daily indoor humidity below 50 per cent will prevent mite population growth and subsequent sleep-disrupting allergens. Even if humidity is lowered, it can take several months for all the allergens to disappear, however.

Noise

People can be awoken by neutral sounds louder than 45 decibels (dB), the equivalent to someone talking quietly (a lawnmower is around 105dB and the threshold for injury to the ear is around 140dB). However, sounds as low as 20dB (below the hearing threshold) can prevent you from falling asleep.

Conversely, continuous background sounds can be soporific

must know

Decibels
Noise is measured in decibels (dB). A 3dB change is detectable but because of the scale used with decibels an increase of 3 means that the noise level has actually doubled.

Noise table

Type of noise	Decibels (dB)
Faintest, audible sounds	0.2–20
TV sound studio, quiet library	20–30
Quiet office	40–50
Conversation	50–60
Primary school classroom, loud radio	60–70
Power drill	85–90
Road drill	100–110
Chainsaw	110–115
Jet aircraft taking off, 25 miles away	140

and it seems that sounds even below 20dB can induce sleepiness – a clear danger for lorry and train drivers. Irregular high-frequency noise can have the opposite effect and be intrusive.

Noise is a problem in many hospitals, particularly in intensive care units. Research has shown that noise in the latter does disturb sleep, and it could be argued that healing processes could be facilitated if natural sleep were promoted. Studies have shown that in neonatal intensive care units, for example, very low birth weight babies sleep more deeply and cry less if quiet hours are introduced. Playing ocean sounds to mask the noise in an intensive care unit has been found to work.

In controlled studies, traffic noise has been shown to increase the time it takes to get to sleep and to lead to greater irritability. Aircraft noise from airports can affect EEG results, showing lighter sleep. However, despite the fact that higher psychiatric hospital admission rates, GP visits and self-reported health problems have been

must know
Vibrations
Vibration can affect sleep just as much as noise. It has been found that even quiet traffic noise of 50dB, when accompanied by vibrations, is more disturbing than when there is just noise. REM sleep is more affected than other stages of sleep. Performance the following day can be impaired.

reported near airports, the effects are highly variable from individual to individual, some being oblivious to the noise levels, others not.

Installing double- or triple-glazing in your home may help, as will wearing ear-plugs, though there is an obvious danger with the latter of possibly life-saving alarms not being heard.

Snoring partners

Many people find snoring amusing, but its long-term effects can be damaging to both the person who snores and their partner. Snoring (covered in more detail on pages 134-6) has been reported to disturb at least 20 per cent of the adult population and has led to numerous social problems ranging from marital disharmony to murder.

A survey using a throat microphone found that 81 per cent of men snored for more than 10 per cent of the night and 22 per cent snored for more than 50 per cent of the night. Other studies have found that women exposed to loud snoring have a higher rate of health complaints, including (not surprisingly) hearing loss!

watch out!

The disadvantage of not seeking help for your snoring problem is that you may be suffering from a more serious sleep breathing disorder: Obstructive Sleep Apnoea (OSA – see page 132).

Although snoring is less prevalent among women, research shows that between 10 and 20 per cent suffer habitual problems and that the incidence increases after the menopause (see page 55).

Snoring is associated with being male. This may be because the anatomy of men and women is different, while the distribution of body fat also predisposes men to snoring. It has also been suggested that women perceive and report snoring more than men. Although there is no universal cure for snoring (possibly because it has so many different anatomical causes), limiting alcohol intake and losing weight may help – research shows there is a clear link between obesity and snoring.

Tranquillizers, sleeping pills and smoking are also all believed to exacerbate the condition.

Temperature

Body temperature is one of the most sensitive markers of the body's biological clock, and can play an important part in sleep. It is lowest when you are asleep in the early morning, peaks in the early evening and can change with age. Studies have shown that sleep onset is almost invariably associated with a decrease in body temperature, ideally of 0.2°C. Conditions have to be right to allow this decrease to take place.

It is impossible to dictate what temperature you should sleep at, since this will depend on a combination of factors such as your own individual temperature, how much you wear in bed, and the type of bed covering you have, but with a bedcover of normal thickness a room temperature of around 16–18°C (about 62–65°F) is about right, though a baby's room should be kept at around 18°C (65°F). An ambient temperature of 12–13°C (53–55°F) will be too low and may adversely affect sleep.

Shivering or sweating may also prevent sleep. A nude person lying on a bed would find a temperature of around 34°C (93°F) compatible with sleep, or 25°C (77°F) with clothes on. To sum up, keep your bedroom cool when you go to bed, but make sure the heating is on by the time you wake up. Cooler temperatures are generally appropriate but extremes should be avoided – overheating may also disturb sleep, possibly with adverse daytime consequences.

want to know more?

Take it to the next level...
- How much is enough? 94
- Keeping a sleep diary? 97
- Knowing yourself 112
- The brain's metronome 16
- The role of melatonin 16

Other sources
- Specialist suppliers of lights, sunrise alarm clocks. See also www.dynamiclighting.philips.com, www.outsidein.co.uk
- To find the perfect mattress, visit www.spineuniverse.com and www.sleepcouncil.org
- To find the right seat on a plane, visit www.seatguru.com
- For advice on managing jet lag, visit www.ba.com/arriveready
- The Health and Safety Executive for safe noise levels has a website: www.hse.gov.uk/noise
- The University of Sydney hosts the international GI database: www.glycemicindex.com

3 Life's journey

Our sleep needs change with age, and as we approach the later stages of life, the sleep patterns of youth may no longer apply. This chapter looks at sleep at every stage of life's journey, from pregnancy and birth to old age. There is also information on childhood sleeping problems and how to deal with them.

Pregnancy, birth and childhood

Pregnancy is a key life stage that can have enormous effects on sleep. This section tells you what to expect in every trimester, and looks at the sleep patterns of babies and children.

The three trimesters

Almost all women have problems sleeping during pregnancy, and even getting comfortable can come to be a major challenge. The nature of the problems change during the pregnancy, which is usually divided into periods of three months: trimesters.

First trimester

Experienced mothers generally plan for more sleep during the first trimester and can get as much as 45–60 minutes more sleep each night than first-time mothers. The extra sleep should probably make them feel more energetic and so can help make pregnancy a more positive experience.

The hormone progesterone is essential for the maintenance of pregnancy and its secretion from the placenta during this time is likely to cause fatigue and earlier sleep onset – this may be why pregnant women feel drowsier now than before pregnancy. But although progesterone has sleep-inducing effects, it can also cause body temperature rises, which can disturb sleep. Laboratory studies have found an increase in total sleep time but poorer quality sleep due to awakening during the night. Progesterone also affects smooth muscle, which causes the increase in visits to the bathroom to urinate during early pregnancy. Body changes also impact on sleep, making it more comfortable for a woman to sleep on her side. Morning sickness (nausea), can affect the latter part of the night.

Second trimester

The second trimester is marked by less tiredness, fatigue and sleep disruption compared to the first. Visits to the toilet tend to go down at this stage, although heartburn may become a problem because of the growing size of the baby, leading to more acid reflux from the stomach during the night. Frightening dreams or nightmares are likely to increase in frequency now, and are experienced by almost three-quarters of mothers. These sometimes involve the baby, but are generally just a magnification of daytime concerns transposed into the dream world.

Third trimester

One study has shown that by the end of pregnancy 97 per cent of women wake an average three times a night; and two-thirds of these wake five or more times a night. Pain associated with the ligaments between the pelvic bones softening and the joints loosening in preparation for the birth, plus the extra weight of the baby affecting daytime posture, contribute to problems sleeping.

Nasal congestion, the increase in abdominal girth and the uterus pressing on the diaphragm can cause snoring in about 30 per cent of women at this stage. Snoring, particularly if associated with breathing pauses (or apnoea, see page 134) can also lead to high blood pressure, particularly if the snoring is coupled with severe daytime sleepiness, headaches and swollen legs. Studies have shown that women

must know

Sleep positions in pregnancy
• Think about your sleep – plan for changes.
• Sleep when you can so that you don't build up a sleep debt (see page 95).
• Consider using a pillow between your knees, with knees and hips bent to reduce pressure on the lower back.
• Sleeping on your side will be the most comfortable position you can adopt. It will also help your kidneys eliminate fluids, preventing swelling in the ankles. Try changing from left to right whenever you can.

who snore during pregnancy are twice as likely to suffer from hypertension (high blood pressure), pre-eclampsia and intra-uterine growth restriction.

A recent survey reported that more than 25 per cent of pregnant women experience Restless Leg Syndrome (RLS – see page 151) during pregnancy, and especially during the third trimester. The reasons for this are not clear, but it may be caused by pressure on the stomach affecting the intake or absorption of iron or other vitamin deficiencies that are associated with pregnancy.

must know

Disturbed sleep

Specific factors that can disturb sleep in pregnancy include:
● back pain
● nocturnal leg cramps
● restricted movement in bed
● heartburn or acid reflux (see page 47)
● anxiety about delivery
● eating during the night
● foetal movements
● nocturia (see page 161)

Sleep disturbances and labour

A recent study of a group of women in their ninth month of pregnancy tested the connection between sleep disturbances in pregnancy and duration of labour and type of delivery. Women who slept less than six hours a night were found to have longer labours, and were 4–5 times more likely to have Caesarean deliveries. Women with severely disrupted sleep also had longer labours, and were 5.2 times more likely to have a Caesarean.

The baby in the womb

By mid-pregnancy it is possible to monitor a baby's brainwaves. Early changes show movements associated with sleep states. By late pregnancy, there are two well-defined sleep states: REM (see page 20) or active sleep, characterized by low-voltage high-frequency brainwave activity and non-Rapid-Eye-Movement (non-REM) or quiet sleep, characterized by high-voltage low-frequency EEG activity. These states account for 95 per cent of brainwave activity. During each state the baby tends to show specific behaviours. Breathing, swallowing, licking, and eye movements generally occur in REM sleep, whereas apnoea (stopping breathing), the absence of eye movements and increased muscle activity occur in non-REM sleep.

It is likely that sleep, or unconsciousness, is the dominant state for at least 95 per cent of the time for the baby.

Babies

Newborn babies can sleep for up to 18 hours a day. For the first few weeks, sleep tends to occur across the 24 hours, with no particularly dominant sleep period, as the baby's natural circadian rhythms are still being developed. It generally takes about six months for sleep to be more concentrated at night.

Sudden Infant Death Syndrome (SIDS)

The first few months of age are the most vulnerable in terms of susceptibility to Sudden Infant Death Syndrome (SIDS), often known as cot death, with the peak of vulnerability being reached at the age of two months. Studies suggest that countries that have adopted and reinforced 'back to sleep campaigns' (where the baby is put to sleep on its back) have seen large falls in the incidence of SIDS deaths.

The benefits of bed sharing

In evolutionary terms, babies sleeping in the same beds as their mothers is normal behaviour. Victorian times saw an increase in the number of babies that slept away from their mothers and this trend continued for a hundred years or so. More recently, the trend has reversed and, in many countries, surveys since the 1990s indicate that the number of mothers sharing their beds with their babies for part or all of the night has doubled (and may be about 50 per cent of nursing mothers). Breastfeeding mothers are three times as likely to share their

must know

Sudden Infant Death Sydrome (SIDS)

In the UK, an average of six babies a week die unexpectedly. SIDS is defined as the sudden death of an infant under one year old and is the most common cause of death in young babies. The incidence of SIDS is increased if:
• babies do not sleep on their backs
• both parents smoke
• soft bedding is used
• a baby under twelve weeks old shares a bed with another child or parents when they are sleeping

beds, or be in the same room as the baby – perhaps not surprisingly, given the convenience – than bottle-feeding mothers. Apart from enhancing contact, night-time baby–mother proximity, whether sleeping in the same bed or within arm's reach, is also associated with reports of less infant crying, more maternal and infant sleep and increased milk supply.

Studies comparing breastfeeding mothers who sleep with or without their babies show that even in the deepest stages of sleep, mothers woke 30 per cent more frequently when they bed shared. Heightened sensitivity and responsiveness increase the chances of reacting to life-threatening events, and studies have shown that when a committed care-giver sleeps in the same room as a baby the chances of that baby dying from SIDS is reduced by 50 per cent.

There is little doubt that bed sharing is a controversial issue. Paediatric research indicates that bed sharing increases risk of SIDS in very young babies, especially if other risk factors are present (see box, page 49). On the other hand, proximity of the baby facilitates breastfeeding. A cot beside the bed might be one solution as it maintains proximity while minimizing disturbance.

Children

Young children will generally sleep for up to twelve hours a night, with daytime naps of between one and three hours a day. By the age of five, the naps will have stopped and the normal sleep requirement will be 10–12 hours a night. This goes down to about ten hours up until the age of twelve.

The importance of routines

Children need and thrive on routines. With younger children, try to maintain set times for daytime naps, and avoid late-afternoon naps that will make them reluctant to go to sleep at bedtime. Establishing a soothing night-time sleep routine as early as possible is essential. Carrying out such activities as bathtime and story-telling at the same time, and in the same order every night will be reassuring to your child, and reinforce the idea that bedtime is approaching. Despite your best efforts, all children resist the idea of going to bed at some point. Don't be tempted to give in just for an easy life – an over-tired child will only cause problems for you the next day.

Bedtime routines can be quite simple. Give your child a bath, help them to put their pyjamas on and brush their teeth. Put them to bed and read a favourite story. Creating a soothing atmosphere before bedtime is important and will help your child to wind down and prepare themselves for sleep.

Tips for putting children to bed

- Develop an evening routine that provides your children with some quality time with you.
- Avoid giving children caffeine-containing foods or drinks in the evening.
- Provide a sleep-conducive environment and reward good night-time behaviour.
- Decide on a bedtime routine and stick to it.
- Put your child to bed while he/she is still awake or drowsy.
- Try not to let your child fall asleep with a drink.
- If not breastfeeding, avoid taking the child into bed for sleep or to settle.

watch out!

There are strong associations made between childhood sleep disorders and problems associated with any disruptive behaviour, lack of concentration or mood swings. Sleep disorders that are caused and maintained by behavioural factors are common in young children, and can have a significant impact on family life.

Children's sleep disorders

Many children suffer from sleep-related disorders. A full list is given on pages 125-6, but two of the most common sleeping problems are described below.

Obstructive Sleep Apnoea (OSA)

Obstructive Sleep Apnoea (OSA – see also page 132) affects about 3 per cent of children, with 8–12 per cent snoring most nights. It occurs most often between the ages of two and eight years, when lymph glands in the throat relative to the upper airway are at their largest. Upper-airway obstruction during sleep should not be attributed solely to large tonsils and adenoids. In fact, in many children these don't cause significant obstruction, and evidence suggests a poor correlation between tonsil size and risk of OSA.

Other factors that may affect the risk of obstruction include altered upper-airway tone, allergic rhinitis, obesity and genetic factors. In adults, overnight OSA is known to have detrimental effects on verbal and non-verbal intelligence, memory, concentration, problem-solving ability and social functioning. It is believed that children can have the same problems, with, in addition, aggression, hyperactivity, inattention, anxiety and lack of confidence.

Nightmares and night terrors

Nightmares are a fairly common childhood occurrence, although the majority of children should grow out of them by the age of around seven. Recurring nightmares can be a sign of stress and anxiety.

Though not classified as a sleep disorder, 46 per cent of parents report difficulties in getting their babies to sleep and find that their babies wake up at night or too early in the morning. Behaviour and behaviour modification techniques can be employed to improve a baby's sleeping pattern, although this can be hard on the parents as it involves what is called the 'controlled

must know

Tooth grinding

Tooth grinding, or bruxism (see page 152), can occasionally occur in up to 50 per cent of children,

Distinguishing between nightmares and night terrors

	Nightmares	Night terrors
Timing	Often later in the night (REM sleep)	Occur once or twice a night in the first 90–180 minutes of sleep (deep sleep)
Age	Common in childhood	Peak 5–7 years
Duration	May take a while to return to sleep	Last 3–5 minutes
Features on awakening	Recall of events frequent in older child, easily comforted, alert on waking	Unresponsive to parents and no recollection. Confusion on waking
Associated features	May be associated with increased breathing, heart rate, sweating. Looking frightened	Invariably associated with increased heart rate, breathing and sweating
Description of event	Wakes crying and responds to comforting	Begins with a few incoherent words or whimpering then screaming
Treatment	Reassurance. If frequent, then check for medical or psychological conditions	Reassurance. The child will not remember the event so the less fuss made the better

crying technique'. The key features of a programme of this nature are:
- the baby should sleep at the same time(s)
- environmental cues for sleep aid the transition to sleep and can be learned, changed and relearned
- well-fed babies are as likely to cry from fatigue as from pain and discomfort
- allowing an infant to fall asleep without a parent
- developing non-parent cues for sleep, e.g. a teddy bear helps the baby learn to sleep without the parent
- consider crying at sleep onset as being caused by tiredness
- leave an infant crying for five minutes before responding. An additional five minutes to the response time is added for any additional visits

There is little doubt that parents have great difficulty in employing this kind of programme but the benefit is that the baby will learn to sleep by itself.

From adolescence to menopause

As the basic cycle of life takes its course, sleep requirements change, in terms of both length and depth. While young adults spend 25 per cent of their time in REM sleep, this figure drops to only 15 per cent in old age.

did you know?

A major cause of sleepiness in adolescents is chronic partial sleep deprivation.

Adolescence and young adulthood

On average, an adolescent needs around eight and a half to nine hours sleep, though this decreases in the late teens. But this is a time of rampant hormones (growth spurts reach their peak now, with high levels of growth hormone being released during sleep) and multi-active lifestyles. The pressures of fitting in homework between active social lives, late nights, holiday jobs and hours spent on the computer, combined with naturally changing and slow biological clocks, means that everything is thrown out of kilter, as late nights merge further and further into daytime hours. About 11 per cent of adolescents suffer from insomnia. The onset of periods in girls is associated with nearly a three-fold increase in insomnia. The monthly rise and fall of hormones in women, coupled with their caring role in most societies and possibly the demands of a career, all collide and impact on sleep.

Irregular hours and erratic lifestyles can persist for some years, but by the twenties and thirties, a general sleeping pattern of around seven and a half hours emerges. However, long commutes for many people, shift work (see page 110), having children and caring for infirm and elderly parents or relatives all erode into sleep time. The demands made by family and work draw on personal and social resources, and can be conflicting. This can lead to negative emotions which disrupt sleep and cause stress both at work and in the family. Stress and general dissatisfaction in turn leads to unhealthy behaviours and poor physical health, with knock-on effects for sleep.

Middle age

Even if seven and a half hours sleep are achieved, this is gradually reduced to an average of seven hours by middle age. It is now that more problems can begin, as increasing weight gain (usually in men) leads to narrowing of the throat, increasing the likelihood of snoring (see page 134). Women hit the menopause with hot flushes and night sweats that invariably lead to disturbed sleep. Middle-aged men who have a collar-size greater than 16, who snore and are sleepy during the day (see page 96) for the Epworth Sleepiness Scale) are likely to suffer from Obstructive Sleep Apnoea (see page 132). OSA has now been linked with increased incidence of heart attacks, strokes (see page 163) and diabetes. If men snoring did not keep women partners awake then the sweating associated with onset of the menopause might! Unfortunately the incidence of snoring at this time also goes up for women.

Old age

Scientists used to think that older people naturally needed less sleep. But the current view is that the poor sleep experienced by older people is a result of the general deterioration of health in old age. The secretion of some hormones like melatonin do

must know

Fatal familial insomnia (FFI)

FFI is a rare hereditary disease caused by a degeneration of the thalamus, resulting in a loss of sleep, hyperactivity of the sympathetic nervous system, disturbed speech and movement, and un-coordinated muscle twitching, all getting progressively worse until death 9–18 months later.

decline, however. Problems with getting to or staying asleep are common in 23–34 per cent of older people and can be associated with chronic medical conditions, psychiatric problems such as depression, chronic pain and the use of sleep medications. Thus in many cases, insomnia is due to some other underlying problem and is not just a consequence of ageing.

Reduced quality of sleep is also a frequent problem. Drowsiness (Stage 1 sleep – see page 18) increases, and is accompanied by an increase in sleep-onset time, early-morning awakenings and difficulties returning to sleep. The reduction in Stage 3 and 4 sleep is a prominent feature of ageing, particularly in men, and is accompanied by a decline in the release of growth hormones. Since growth hormones are involved in the regulation of non-REM sleep, it has been suggested that the two are linked. (This decline starts at around 30 years of age.) Studies investigating the role of 24-hour rhythms in age-related sleep changes indicate that older people have difficulty in sustaining sleep at particular times during the day. In strictly controlled laboratory studies, older subjects of 64–74 years of age were found to wake up earlier. Increasing age was associated with a lower percentage of light exposure during the night and with a higher percentage of light exposure in the morning, suggesting that circadian rhythms (see page 14) are speeded up in the middle years of life.

Some age-related sleeping problems

The increased incidence of Obstructive Sleep Apnoea (OSA – see page 132) with age means that a number of symptoms like headaches and nocturia (see page

Sleeptime strategies for the elderly

● Review your caffeine and alcohol intake (see page 30), as both can have a more powerful effect with age.

● Stick to a regular waking time, however difficult this may be.

● Make sure your room temperature (see page 43) is correct – we get more sensitive to temperature as we age.

● Be positive. A 2003 poll carried out by the American National Sleep Foundation found a direct link between positive outlook and good sleep in the elderly.

● Make sure you do not have a sleep-related disorder (see Chapter 6).

● Be prepared to go to your doctor and discuss alternatives if you are taking a medication that is affecting your sleep.

● Change your schedule to accommodate the change in your sleeping habits.

58) can be be caused or exacerbated by the breathing disorder. Treating the apnoea, which is increasingly associated with hypertension, coronary artery disease and diabetes, is the priority. Key sleep-disrupting problems during ageing are shown above.

Hormonally related sleep-disordered breathing

This is often associated with the menopause. It is believed that female hormones, and progesterone in particular, may play a role in protecting pre-menopausal women from sleep-disordered breathing. As these hormones decrease, sleep-disordered breathing increases.

Visual impairment

Visual impairment is a common and disabling disorder in the elderly. Its prevalence increases from

must know

Morvan's Fibrillary Chorea

This is a rare disease marked by the onset of severe insomnia and hyperactivity of the sympathetic nervous system similar to FFI (see box on opposite page). It is also associated with cramps and muscle twitching and is characterized by spontaneous remission in 90 per cent of cases with progression to death in only 10 per cent of cases.

18 per cent in men and 26 per cent in women of ages 65–69 years to 31 per cent in men and 47 per cent of women of age 80 years or over. Poor sleep, frequent awakening and difficulty in falling asleep afterwards all increase in visually impaired elderly persons, and these in turn result in daytime sleepiness and a need for napping. As the retina ages, the input into the biological clock also probably diminishes, partly accounting for the earlier sleep onset and early-morning awakening. This further complicates the health problems found in older people.

must know

Sleep and death
A survey carried out by the American Cancer Society found that longer sleeping hours related to significantly higher mortality rates; elderly people sleeping between 3.5 and 4.5 hours had lower mortality levels than those sleeping more than 7.5 hours! The reason is not clear, but the higher mortality rates may be due to an underlying sleep disorder.

Headaches

Approximately 10 per cent of women and 5 per cent of men at age 70 experience severe recurrent or constant headaches that can lead to disturbed sleep. Headaches in the elderly can be migrainous, tension, cluster or hypnic (see pages 157–60), but secondary causes such as circulatory problems, glaucoma, tumours, haemorrhages or side-effects from medication are also possible. Sleep apnoea may also cause or exacerbate headache. One study of 37 females aged 65–94 years found a positive correlation between snoring and the frequency of nightmares and morning headaches. Nightmares and morning head-aches were also linked to one another. Snoring was also associated with the number of brief awakenings during sleep and with increased body weight.

Nocturia

Another problem that elderly people can suffer from is nocturia (frequent night-time urination). Sufficient sleep is known to inhibit night-time urination, so any impairment in sleep is likely to lead to nocturia.

In addition to the above, the following can also afflict the sleep of the elderly:

- immobility
- falling
- medications
- swallowing
- nocturnal cramps

Death and his brother sleep

It is a curious fact that sleep and death are related. Most sleep-related death is caused by drowsiness leading to accidents – car accidents in particular – but there are also associations between sleep and mortality in general. Mortality rate starts to increase in the late hours of the night, around the time that REM sleep is most prevalent, and continues to rise to a maximum between 8 a.m. and 10 a.m. in the morning. As REM is a time when the body's physiology is less well regulated, it is possible that people who are prone to either heart attacks or strokes find themselves succumbing. It is also possible that the relative inactivity caused by sleep increases the thickness or cohesiveness of the blood so that the extra work imposed on the heart upon awakening and sudden movement is enough to cause a catastrophic event.

want to know more?

Take it to the next level...
- Breathing and relaxation techniques 68
- Clocks, cycles and rhythms 14
- Conditions that can affect sleep 154
- Melatonin 16
- Sleep-related breathing disorders 132
- The stages of sleep 18

Other sources
- National Sleep Foundation: www.sleepfoundation.org
- NHS Direct, www.nhsdirect.nhs.uk
- US National Library of Medicine: www.nlm.nih.gov/medlineplus/sleepdisorders
- University of Maryland Medical Center: www.umm.edu/sleep/sleep_dis_child

4 How to sleep better

In our 'here and now' society, sleeping pills can offer a quick-and-easy fix. But although they may provide a temporary answer, they won't help in the long term – and many of them have side-effects. With practical suggestions on how to improve your sleeping environment, encouragement on getting into good sleeping habits, and simple relaxation exercises and alternative therapies, this chapter offers you healthier and longer-lasting solutions.

Sleep hygiene

The rather strange term 'sleep hygiene' is one that is often used in sleep medicine today, and refers to environmental and lifestyle issues that can affect sleep. Applied correctly, sleep hygiene can play a key role in getting a good night's sleep.

The basic essentials for good 'sleep hygiene' are to try to have regular times for sleeping, to avoid eating or drinking anything that might disturb sleep and to be as comfortable as possible. That comfort should be physical (the right pillow, mattress, duvet, temperature, light, heat, humidity and noise) and mental (feeling-well, carefree, safe and relaxed).

Top tips for good sleep hygiene

- Avoid alcohol, tobacco or caffeine – especially at night.
- Try to avoid exciting or emotionally upsetting activities too close to bedtime.
- Do not have a television in your room. Your bedroom should be kept exclusively for sleep (and sex).
- Try not to read in bed.
- Make sure you have a comfortable bed with a good mattress and pillows.
- Block out any excessive noise with ear-plugs or, if necessary, double-glazing.
- Block out light with heavy curtains.
- Make sure your room is reasonably cool.
- Try to go to bed and get up at the same time every day.
- Establish regular wind-down techniques such as having a warm, scented bath before going to bed.
- Do not eat a heavy meal late at night.
- Avoid rich, fatty or spicy foods.

Is your bedroom conducive to a good night's sleep?

If you answer 'yes' to three or more of these questions, you may need to rethink your sleeping space.

Questions	Yes	No
● Do you have one lightsource in the bedroom?	☐	☐
● Do you have a TV in your bedroom?	☐	☐
● Do you use your bedroom as an office as well as a place to sleep?	☐	☐
● Is your bedroom cluttered?	☐	☐
● Does your bedroom overlook a noisy road?	☐	☐
● Do you have see-through curtains over the windows in your room?	☐	☐
● Do you wake up with aches and pains, or feeling stiff?	☐	☐
● Do you often have a crick in your neck when you wake up?	☐	☐
● Do you suffer from frequent backache?	☐	☐

must know

Bedtime routines
It is important to establish a regular bedtime routine, if possible. Your internal bodyclock is synchronized to its regular sleeping/waking routine every night and morning, so even minor changes can have a negative effect. Both brain and body need to settle down to sleep and for some people this means a wind-down routine needs to start an hour or so before bed. For others it may only need to be 30 minutes, or just a leisurely time spent in the bathroom.

A comfortable sleeping environment

Creating a comfortable sleeping environment is a crucial aspect of sleep hygiene. In Chapter 2 (page 38) we looked at the importance of temperature, light, humidity and noise in the bedroom, all of which will have an impact upon your quality of sleep. But attending to these factors alone might not be enough. You may also need to consider changing more specific aspects of your sleeping environment, such as your mattress and pillows.

Beds

You will spend a third of your life asleep, so getting the right mattress is crucial. If you wake up with aches and pains that go away within a few hours of their own accord, it is almost certainly the surface you're sleeping on that is causing the problem.

Should I buy a bed with a hard or soft mattress? This is probably the question most frequently asked by bed-buyers. Up until recently, the received view has been that hard mattresses are a better option than soft, because they offer better support for the back. But opinion is now more generally divided. Hard mattresses may indeed provide support, but their contact points can sometimes be limited and may touch your body in specific areas that are sensitive, causing pain as constant pressure is applied. Soft mattresses, on the other hand, provide continual body contact, but the lack of support can cause the neck and spine to sag, resulting in muscle tension and pain.

Rather than thinking in terms of hard and soft, therefore, it may be more helpful to think in terms of mattresses that are *firm*. The level of firmness should relate to your body weight (the heavier you are, the firmer the mattress should be) and the mattress should,

watch out!

If you sleep with your partner, buy the biggest bed you can. Most standard double beds give both partners less space than a single bed each would.

Beds – a historical perspective

• 17th century: Louis XIV was extremely fond of staying in bed, and would often hold court in the royal bedroom. He is said to have owned 413 beds in all!

• 19th century: writer Charles Dickens believed that the direction a bed pointed was important for good sleep – head pointing north, feet south – and therefore carried a compass on his journeys so that he could align his bed properly. In those days people believed that the flow of magnetic currents from north to south would benefit the sleeper if it went straight through their body.

• 20th century: politician Winston Churchill liked to sleep in the nude. Like Franklin, he liked to have two beds, so that he could move to one with unwrinkled sheets when he had rumpled the sheets of the one he was sleeping in!

ideally, distribute pressure evenly across your body (important for healthy circulation) and make uninterrupted contact with it.

Make sure that you change your mattress every ten years, as any regular use after this can lead to deterioration. You can choose from a variety of mattress 'fillings': internal spring unit (pocket-sprung, continuous springing or open coil), latex, foam or cotton. Many manufacturers recommend spring units: the higher the spring count, the better (and more expensive!). In recent years, 'memory foam' mattresses which adapt to your shape and weight have become popular. Finally, don't be afraid

did you know?
The expression 'sleep tight' comes from the 16th and 17th centuries, when mattresses were placed on top of ropes that needed regular tightening.

must know

Buying sheets
Where possible, choose natural fabrics that will let your skin breathe. For a really soft and comfortable feel, linen is best, even though it is more expensive. Look for linen with a high thread density - it will feel softer on your skin.

to try different ones out in the shop before you buy. This could well be one of the most important purchases you ever make.

Ergonomics experts from Cornell University, USA, have given the following guidelines for choosing a mattress. An ideal mattress should be:

- designed to conform to the spine's natural curves and to keep the spine in alignment
- made in such a way that it distributes pressure evenly across the body
- designed to minimize the transfer of movement from one sleeping partner to the other

If in doubt, contact the Sleep Council (see want to know more? on page 91).

Pillow support posture

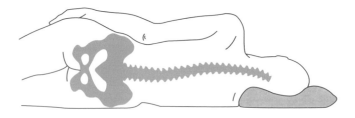

Poor sleep position posture

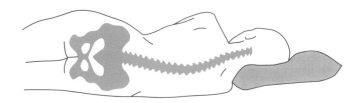

Ideal posture

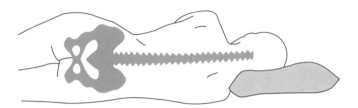

Pillows

One of the most common causes of sleeping problems is poor body alignment in bed. Buying the right pillow will help. Pillows should support your neck as well as your head and maintain a straight line between your neck and spine. There are many special pillows available now with built-in head and neck support that should do this successfully, but if in doubt, consult an osteopath or chiropractor.

An ideal pillow should:
- maintain the natural alignment of your spine
- be easily adjustable to fit your neck and head contours
- support your head
- maintain a straight line between your neck and spine
- be hypoallergenic (for house dust sufferers)

must know
Beauty sleep
To stop getting skin creases from pillows and sheets, actresses have known since the early days of cinema that sleeping on silk pillow-cases and sheets prevents this from happening. Drinking water and using night-time moisturizing lotions also help avoid creasing in the morning.

Breathing and relaxation techniques

Sleepless nights can often lead to a vicious circle where the very anxiety about not sleeping can exacerbate the problem. Before reaching out for that sleeping pill, try the deep breathing and relaxation techniques below and see the difference.

must know

Room temperature
Your body temperature will drop soon after you exercise because the blood vessels near your skin will open up to release heat. As part of the process of going to sleep involves lowering body temperature, it is helpful to have a slightly cool room (around 17°C) to enable this to happen.

The art of relaxing

Chronic insomnia can become a self-perpetuating cycle in which anxiety about not sleeping can become worse than the problem itself. As the anxiety increases, muscles tense up and sleep becomes impossible, increasing the anxiety again. And so the cycle continues, seemingly with no end. It is in this kind of situation that deep breathing, meditation and relaxation exercises come into their own. Used correctly, they can help to relax the mind or the body – and, in some cases, both.

The three most beneficial ways you can use breathing for relaxation are in meditation, deep breathing and progressive muscle relaxation. None of these techniques are mutually exclusive; they can be used individually or together. The best thing to do is to learn each one separately and practise them at least once or twice a day for about a week in order to master them properly, then use them as coping strategies during the night if you can't sleep. Although deep breathing is an art in itself, learning how to breathe properly is the key to using all three relaxation techniques.

The art of breathing

There are a variety of breathing techniques, most of which have developed from Eastern meditative and yogic practices. It may sound strange to talk in terms of 'techniques' for something we do every second of the day, but, curiously, in the West, none of us seem to know how to breathe properly. In any group of Westerners who are asked to take a deep breath, it is striking to see that only their chests rise as they breathe in (shallow breathing). In a similar group from the East, their stomachs and abdomens will rise as well as their chests, indicating that they are breathing deeply. Deep-breathing techniques can easily be learned, however.

Deep breathing

The good thing about deep breathing is that it is completely under your individual control. Although the effects of deep breathing are chiefly psychological, by doing it you also bring about a physiological change on the body itself, because slowing down the breathing will also slow down your heart rate.

When you get anxious, a couple of things happen: (1) the stress stimulates the body to go into 'fight or flight' (see page 36), in which heart rate and respiration speed up; and (2) the brain interprets this response as a cause of stress, and puts the body back into fight or flight again, thereby increasing the anxiety, and so on, in the vicious cycle described above. Deep breathing will break part of the cycle by producing a physiological response in both the heart and respiration rate, which in turn will help to calm the mind.

must know
Breathing and meditation
Exhalation is very important in breathing exercises, as the end of each breath signals the point of letting go of anxious thoughts. The moment of silence between breathing in and breathing out is the goal that most meditators aim for.

How to do deep breathing

Lie on your back, legs outstretched, with one hand on your chest and the other on your abdomen. Breathe in slowly through your nostrils, and try to feel the breath moving through your chest. Feel your chest rise, and as it does so let the breath continue to enter your body, and let your stomach and abdomen push upwards towards the ceiling until your lungs are as full of air as possible. Ideally, the hand on your abdomen will now be higher than the one on your chest. Pause for a moment, and let the air out of your stomach and abdomen first, and then your chest. As you breathe out, the muscles generally start to relax and your

must know

Deep breathing

It can sometimes be difficult to feel the movement of your diaphragm if you are lying on your back. An alternative might be to lie on your stomach with your legs stretched out, your toes pointing outwards and your arms folded under your chest in such a way that your chest doesn't touch the floor.

Abdominal breathing

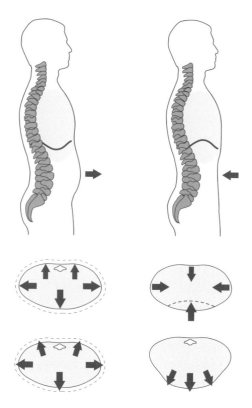

jaw should be unclenched. Try this exercise during the day, and repeat at night if necessary.

Breathing variations

There are several variations on breathing techniques. Here are two:

1. Put your finger over your left nostril, and breathe in through your right one, then put your finger over the right one and breathe out through the left one.

2. Count your breaths. Inhale and exhale (count 'one'), inhale and exhale (count 'two') and carry on up to a count of four, then start again. You may inevitably find that stray thoughts and worries get in the way of your counting. If this happens, return to 'one' and continue.

Meditation

Breathing is closely associated with meditation. The world's most important ancient religions – Buddhism, Hinduism, Islam, Judaism, early Christianity, Jainism, Shinto and Taoism – have been based on teaching their followers to turn their minds inwards as a means of gaining inner peace and happiness. It is only in relatively recent Western history that the practice of contemplation or meditation has been lost, with the consequence that many people now look towards the East, where these practices are still observed.

So what is meditation?

Meditation is a state in which the mind is freed from its usual clutter. An often used analogy is that the mind in meditation is rather like a sky where there are no clouds to obscure the blueness. Extending this analogy, to be in a state of meditation is to experience a mind that is unclouded by thinking, feeling, prejudice, etc. One way of letting go of these feelings is to close your eyes and imagine a series of boxes that have labels on them – Anxiety, Unhappy Memories, New Ideas, a Pending Task, Regret, or whatever, and then to let the unwelcome thoughts run through your body and identify them. The idea is that you create a box for each of these distractions, and as each one appears, you put it in its box and leave it there. You can always come back to the boxes later.

How to meditate

The meditation described here has two phases: the initial, preparatory stage, when you slowly let your mind drift in preparation for the meditation; and the meditation itself, which is known as a breath meditation. You can make it last for anything from ten minutes to half an hour.

must know

Yoga

Hatha yoga comes from the words ha meaning 'sun' and tha meaning 'moon'. The slower breath through the right nostril represents the 'sun' breath and the flow of the breath through the left nostril is the 'moon'. Breath regulation is central to hatha yoga as it is believed to bring about the harmonization of the forces of the sun and the moon.

Preparation

1. Start by finding a place where you can sit undisturbed and in comfort. You ideally need to be in a position where you can feel relaxed without falling asleep, but as upright as possible. Sitting cross-legged on the floor is ideal.

2. Rest your hands on your legs, and try to settle into a comfortable position.

3. Take a moment to look around the room and notice everything as if it were new.

4. When you feel completely settled, close your eyes, take several deep breaths and feel the air rush in and out, as if you were sighing. Try to enjoy the feeling of letting go. Let your shoulders relax and drop, and at the same time feel your spine lengthening.

5. Slowly let your breath settle back into its normal rhythm.

6. Become aware of your body. Try to relax the areas that are tense.

Breath meditation

1. Settle down comfortably, close your eyes and start by taking a few deep breaths.

2. As you exhale, let go and feel the tensions in your body disappear. If you still find you are having tense feelings, breathe into them and try letting them go.

3. Feel your spine lengthen as if somebody has attached a string to your head and is pulling it a little.

4. Relax your face muscles and let your tongue become relaxed as you start to breathe more deeply.

> **did you know?**
> Yogis sleep on their left side so as to leave their right nostril uppermost. It is meant to make their sleep more refreshing.

5. Start to feel the breath coming in and out through your nose, then, as your breathing gets deeper, feel the breath entering your throat, chest and lower abdomen.

6. Try to breathe a little more deeply through your abdomen, following the breath as you breathe in and out. As you breathe out, try to let go completely.

7. Try to pinpoint the moment where you stop inhaling and are about to exhale, and let that moment between breathing in and out be a moment of exquisite silence. As you breathe out, let any remaining tensions go, then slow your breathing down.

8. When you want to come out of your meditation, listen to what is around you, tilt your head back a little, then your hands and your body. Open your eyes, look around. Return to the starting point.

Yoga

Yoga is an ancient form of exercise developed more than 5000 years ago in India, where it is still widely practised. It is believed to have both mental and physical benefits, reducing stress and increasing suppleness, both of which can benefit sleep. It can involve special physical postures (asanas), forms of breathing control (pranayamas), maintenance of silence (mouna),meditation (dhyana) and visual focusing exercises (tratakas).

In the West, yoga is known mainly as a method of stretching and exercising, with some meditation and breathing control. But in India it is connected with the Hindu religion. For Hindu mystics the main aim of yoga is a union between the universal and individual beings. In fact the word 'yoga' means union. The best-known form of yoga is hatha yoga (see page 72). This is the form that is most widely practised in the West, but for true Eastern practitioners it is not considered to be yoga at all but, rather, a collection or system of exercises that can serve other forms of yoga (see box left).

(see page 72)

must know

Types of yoga

There are many different types of yoga, each based on a different form of harmony or union. Some of the most important forms are as follows:

- Jnana (union by knowledge)
- Bhakti (union by love and devotion)
- Karma (union by action and service)
- Mantra (union by voice and sound)
- Yantra (union by vision and form)
- Kundalini (union by raising spiritual consciousness)
- Tantric (union that harnesses sexual energy)
- Hatha (union by mastery of the body, principally breath)
- Raja (union by mental mastering)

Progressive muscle relaxation and autogenics

Progressive muscle relaxation and autogenics both work on the principle of gradually relaxing separate groups of muscles. But while in progressive muscle relaxation each muscle in the body is relaxed by doing specific physical exercises, in autogenics the relaxation is visualized rather than actually carried out. Autogenics can be particularly useful for elderly people, who find it difficult or uncomfortable to contract certain muscles.

Progressive muscle relaxation

1. Start with your feet, concentrating on one foot first (it doesn't matter which). Tighten your toes, then bend them, stretch and relax. Extend the toes, stretch the muscles, keep them stretched and then relax.

2. Move both feet so that your heels are pointing away from you. Hold and relax.

3. Stretch your feet upwards, your heels raised off the ground. Hold and relax. Repeat.

4. Feel your feet and toes beginning to relax. Your leg should already be starting to relax too. Feel the warmth as your muscles relax.

5. Pull one foot up and hold it in position until you feel slight tension in your calves and thighs. Hold until the tension makes your muscles feel they are working hard and think about what's happening. They are beginning to feel a little cramped...there's a burning sensation. Relax and feel the blood going through your muscles. Repeat with the other foot.

6. Stretch out your feet and feel the other muscles tightening. Concentrate on your feet, then your calves, shins and thighs. Once you start to feel your muscles have had enough, relax. Now compare the way the muscles in your feet feel to how they were when you started. They should be much more relaxed.

7. Keeping your breathing regular, take one deep breath and as you exhale, think 'one'. Breathe in, and as you exhale, think 'two'. Breathe in, and as you exhale, think 'three'. Breathe in, and as you exhale, think 'four'.

8. Move on and concentrate on your thighs, following the same principles as on the feet. Work on the rest of the muscles on your body, concentrating on your abdomen, stomach, chest, then your hands and arms, back, neck, jaw, cheeks, brow, scalp, so that you've worked all the way up your body.

9. You are now warm, comfortable and relaxed. You won't need to finish the routine. Just let yourself drift off when you're feeling sleepy.

Diet and nutrition

Adopt healthy eating routines, especially if your sleep diary (page 97) has shown that your sleep problems are food-related.

Nutrients for healthy sleep

The amino acids, vitamins and minerals shown below are important for promoting healthy sleep. Eat them in natural sources, rather than as supplements, if you can:

B-vitamins: These are the vitamins that are most closely associated with sleep, possibly because they are involved in the control of tryptophan (see right) and other sleep-inducing amino acids.

B3 (niacin or niacinamide) has been found to be useful in insomnia and depression.

Sources: red meat, chicken and turkey, salmon, tuna, mackerel, wholewheat, wheatgerm, dried apricots

B6 (pyridoxine) is a required cofactor for the absorption of magnesium (see right), protein and essential fatty acids. It aids in the production of the brain chemical, serotonin (see page 17).

Sources: wholegrains, wheatgerm, potatoes, watercress, bananas, walnuts

B12 (cobalamine) has been found to be useful in relieving fatigue and anxiety, which can be a major cause of insomnia. It can also amplify the effect of melatonin (see page 16).

Sources: dairy products, seafood, eggs, meat

watch out!

Caffeine has the biggest effect on sleep (see page 30). Remember that it is not only coffee and tea that contain caffeine - it is also present in alcohol. Drinking too much alcohol before you go to bed will almost certainly disturb your sleep (see page 30 and box opposite). Nicotine is also detrimental to a good night's sleep (see page 37).

Iron: Iron deficiency has been strongly associated with Restless Leg Syndrome (RLS - see page 15), which is a major cause of sleep disruption. Note: iron supplements should not be taken in excess.

Sources: meat, poultry, liver, spinach

Magnesium: Magnesium is often called Nature's tranquillizer and deficiencies are associated with early-morning awakening. Supplements have been shown to have a positive effect.
Sources: avocados, wheatgerm, bananas, green leafy vegetables, nuts and seeds, wholegrains

Tryptophan: An essential amino acid, there have been health scares over its use as a supplement, and over-the-counter forms have been banned, but it is perfectly harmless when taken in food and drink.
Sources: turkey, bananas, dairy products, almonds, cabbage, kidney beans, oats, spinach, wheat, poultry, eggs, red meats, tofu and other soy products.

Zinc and calcium: These have all been associated with improvements in sleep.
Sources: brewer's yeast, dairy products, oats, pumpkin seeds

Good sleep suppers and bedtime snacks

Stagger your meals so that you eat little and often, and avoid over-eating at night. If you must eat late, foods that are high in carbohydrates and calcium and low in protein are best.

Snacks:
- wholegrain cereals with milk
- oat biscuits
- hazelnuts and tofu
- hummus and wholewheat pitta bread

Meals:
- scrambled eggs with cheese
- tofu stif-fry
- chicken or turkey with vegetables
- pasta with parmesan cheese

Alternative therapies

Recent years have seen an increase in the popularity of alternative therapies. Although there is no scientific evidence that they work, many people find them useful for treating mild sleep problems. Below is an A–Z of the most popular forms.

must know

Sleep remedies
Aspirin increases slow wave sleep and has been found to work on some insomniacs who wake late in the night. The effect lasts only a couple of nights, however, so it should only be tried occasionally. Read the warnings on the label – aspirin is not safe for everyone!

Acupuncture

Acupuncture is a Chinese system of medicine in which needles are used to stimulate certain points in the body, known as meridians, to increase the flow of *chi* (or life force) into different parts of the body. It is useful in relieving pain, which can often cause insomnia, as well as in promoting relaxation. There are often specific acupuncture 'points' for each condition. A Chinese medical practitioner's reasoning will determine the precise points that are used, but Sp6, K3 and H7 are often focused on to treat insomnia.

Alexander technique

Alexander technique attempts to identify and release areas of unwanted muscle tension by correcting body misalignment. It was developed by Australian actor and teacher F. Matthias Alexander (1869-1955), who developed a method of voice training that was based on respiratory control. It can be carried out on a one-to-one basis or in a group. See page 188 for a qualified practitioner. The alexander technique is particularly useful for relieving postural problems and imbalances that can often cause sleeplessness.

Aromatherapy

Aromatherapy relies on the use of essential oils, extracted from flowers, herbs and trees, to promote

Good aromatherapy sleep oils

Bergamot (*Citrus bergamia*)	Refreshing and uplifting after a stressful day
Clary sage (*Salvia sclarea*)	Relaxing and an antidepressant. Good for stress and depression
Frankincense (*Boswellia carterii*)	Relieves fear and anxiety
Lavender (*Lavandula officinalis*)	The best-known and most popular oil for sleep problems
Roman chamomile (*Anthemis nobilis*)	Soothing, relaxing and calming

health and wellbeing. The idea is that the oils stimulate the olfactory organs, which are linked to the parts of the brain that cause specific emotions. Aromatherapy oils can either be used for massage (in which case they will mostly have to be mixed with a 'carrier' oil such as almond) or added to the bath. Some of the most popular oils are listed above.

Bach flower remedies

These were invented by Dr Edward Bach at the turn of the 20th century. Bach believed that the remedies derived from wild flowers and spring water provided a subtle energy form that was effective in treating emotional disharmony. The remedies are prepared by picking fresh flowers and placing them on the surface of a bowl of water where they are left for several hours in the sun. The essences are then distilled and mixed with water and tiny amounts of alcohol. Specific remedies are made up for specific personality traits and can be self-administered in liquid form. The main one associated with insomnia is White Chestnut (for an overactive mind that stops you sleeping).

Baths

Hot baths increase slow-wave sleep, and may be generally conducive to sleep. It is not clear why they work, but it may be something to do with the fact that the hot water opens up blood vessels, which helps you to cool down. Foot baths may also be helpful. One technique is to have two foot baths, one filled with warm-to-hot water, the other with cold water. Place one foot in each for a few minutes, then change over.

Biofeedback

Biofeedback is a form of headache treatment that uses the electronic feedback of hand temperature and/or muscle tension to teach patients deep relaxation. Acquiring and regularly practising these skills has been shown to often reduce the frequency and severity of both migraine and tension-type headaches that can disrupt sleep (see pages 157–60).

Biorhythm calculations

In this case the word 'biorhythm' refers to three theoretical rhythms that were first identified at the turn of the 20th century by an associate of Sigmund Freud, Dr Wilhelm Fleiss. After examining medical records, he concluded that a solar cycle (dominant in men) influenced physical health and a lunar cycle (dominant in women) influenced emotions. In the 1920s, a third cycle controlling intellectual function was postulated by Austrian mathematician Professor Alfred Teltscher after he observed fluctuations in academic performance in his students. Biorhythms are calculated using birth date. The physical cycle, affecting strength, stamina, coordination, immunity and sex drive, follows a 23-day rhythm. A 28-day cycle governs mood and creativity, the theory goes, and memory and concentration run on a 33-day rhythm. If charted, individuals can identify days when they are particularly vulnerable and days when they can expect optimal functioning. These biorhythms are completely different to the biological clock rhythms that have been described earlier in this book (see page 14), and there is little scientific support for their use.

Chinese medicine

Apart from acupuncture, traditional Chinese remedies include herbalism, using a wide range of plant remedies such as jujube seeds and fleece-flower (see also Herbs, overleaf). An ancient remedy known as *suanzaorentang* was originally described in an old Chinese text, *Kin-Kue-Yao-Lueh,* as being good for patients with muscle weakness, irritability and insomnia. It has been tested using conventional Western techniques and preliminary observations indicate anxiety-relieving properties. The science involved a controlled clinical trial comparing various doses of suanzaorentang with diazepam. Both had similar anxiety-relieving properties, but unlike diazepam, which impairs daytime performance, suanzaorentang caused no such impairment. To find a properly accredited practitioner of Chinese medicine, contact the Register of Chinese Herbal Medicine. See also Useful addresses, pages 188–9.

must know
Finding a practitioner
When finding any type of alternative health practitioner, always make sure they have the correct professional qualifications and are registered with an organization. Official societies for each therapy are available on the relevant websites. See also the Useful addresses section in this book (pages 188–9).

Electrosleep therapy

This therapy uses electricity or electromagnetic radiation to promote sleep and has been around almost as long as electricity itself. Early research found various problems with the methods that were used, but recent research using an electric spoon that is placed in the mouth has produced surprisingly good results. However, high levels of placebo (dummy or blank treatment) response in insomnia trials creates a problem in assessing the real utility of this method either to promote sleep or for relaxation.

Feng shui

This increasingly popular system of thought is said to be the practice of living harmoniously with the energy of the surrounding environment, which naturally leads to the art of placement, not only of buildings, but of everything within them. Traditionally taught and practised in the Far East, it was originally used as a method of determining where to site graves. It was also used to decide when and where to build a home or community.

Hands-on healing

Hands-on healing and other forms of faith healing work on the basis that the mind guides the body, and faith-healers empower the mind, allowing it to channel its energy to either improve body function or make the body feel better. There are various methods, practices and techniques, such as cranosacral therapy, myofascial release, muscle energy technique, visceral manipulation, strain and counterstrain, and massage.

must know

Feng shui in your bedroom
According to feng shui, the layout of your bedroom is all-important for a good night's sleep. The idea is that the *chi* (energy) in your environment should be harmonized to best advantage.

Herbs

Herbal preparations usually have considerable folklore associated with them to attest to their efficacy and are generally thought by the public to be safe because they are natural. This is a false premise, however. Poisonous mushrooms, to take an example, are natural but are definitely not safe. The active ingredients of many herbal preparations are unknown, and often there is no guarantee that a particular crop is a good one. Occasionally herbs actually contain ingredients that are used in sleeping pills and tranquillizers. A classic example of this is valerian, which forms the basis of Valium-based drugs! While it is possible to buy medicinal herbs easily and the right to grow and consume these in England has existed since Henry VIII's time, it

Top feng shui tips

1. Ideally, the bedroom should be as far away as possible from the front door.

2. Avoid positioning your bed between the door and any windows.

3. Position your bed so that you can see the door from where you sleep. This will give you a deep sense of inner security.

4. Position your bed as far away from the door as possible.

5. Avoid sleeping with your head close to a window as your *chi* will dissipate through the window and make you feel more tired on awakening.

6. If you have a bathroom, toilet or shower leading off from your bedroom, make sure that the door is always shut while you are asleep.

7. Make sure that you have a strong headboard to help you protect and recharge your *chi* while you are asleep.

8. Make sure all bedside tables have rounded edges and not square to prevent 'cutting' *chi* being focused towards the occupants.

9. Ceiling beams above the bed are a feng shui nightmare, as they can be a source of 'cutting' *chi*. Paint the beams so that they blend in with the ceiling or drape fabric over them.

10. Use soft lighting and avoid ceiling lamps directly over your bed.

11. Use pastel colours.

12. Avoid sleeping with your image visible in a mirror. The worst scenario of all is a mirror at the foot of your bed.

is probably wise to consider visiting a qualified herbalist to get the correct individual herb or mixture.

Below is a list of herbs that are thought to have some beneficial effects on sleep or sleeplessness:

Californian poppy (*Eschscholzia californica* – Papaveraceae)
The euphoriant effect of the poppy plant was reported in ancient Sumerian records around 4000 years ago. The dried aerial parts are used as a sedative and hypnotic and it has the reputation for being a non-addictive alternative to the opium poppy. Traditionally Native Americans have used it for colic pains and to calm over-excitable children.

Chamomile, Garden (*Anthemis nobilis* – Compositae); Chamomile, German (*Matricaria chamomilla* – Compositae)
The flowers are reputed to have multiple actions but are regarded as mild sedatives that can help muscle spasms, anxiety and insomnia. There is some scientific evidence that chamomile extract may have a sleep-inducing activity. The dried flowers are frequently use in herbal teas.

must know
Good herbal remedies for sleep
• Cider vinegar and honey in hot water.
• Teas made from catnip, fennel, melissa or rosemary.

Hops (*Humulus lupulus* – Cannabaceae)
The flower is used widely for the treatment of sleeplessness and is also recommended for anxiety and stress. It is claimed to act as a tranquillizer and is also said to decrease the desire for alcohol! No formal comparisons have been made, but it has been suggested that hops induce sleep more rapidly than valerian. Herbalists advise that hops should not be used if depression is present.

Jamaican dogwood (*Piscidia erythrina* – Leguminosae)
The bark of this plant is collected in vertical strips from trees

growing in the Caribbean, Mexico and Texas. It is regarded as a strong remedy for sleeplessness, particularly when this is caused by pain. Scientific evidence suggests it is a cross between a sleeping agent and an anxiety-reliever.

Lady's slipper (*Cypripedium pubescens* – Orchidaceae)
Lady's slipper is also known as American valerian. Its root is widely used for the treatment of stress, emotional tension and anxiety, especially anxiety associated with sleeplessness.

Lavender (*Lavandula officinalis* – Labiatae)
The flowers are claimed to have an antidepressant and anti-spasmodic action. Lavender is believed to be beneficial in depressive states and may improve sleep in the elderly.

Mullein (*Verbascum thapsus* – Scrophulariaceae)
The leaves of this herb are said to reduce pain, infection and bleeding and are used to stimulate the respiratory system. They are also used as a sleep aid.

Oats (*Avena sativa* – Poaceae)
Long used to treat nervous exhaustion and 'weakness of the nerves', oats are rich in body-building nutrients such as calcium, zinc (see page 77) and vitamins. A tincture of the grains and seeds is a useful remedy for relieving stress, anxiety and insomnia.

Passionflower (*Passiflora incarnata* – Passifloraceae)
Passiflora seeds several thousand years old have been discovered at archaeological sites in North America, indicating that these fruits were highly valued by the indigenous population living there at that time. This group of herbs consists of about 500 species, which grow mainly in the temperate and tropical regions of the New World. The dried leaves are used for

treating intransigent insomnia. The infusions and tinctures are also said to have a role in Parkinson's Disease (see page 162).

Peppermint (*Mentha piperita* – Lamiaceae)
The peppermint herb has been used as a digestive aid for the stomach, a decongestant, an anaesthetic and a germicide, and is believed to be a useful remedy for the common cold. Peppermint is said to promote relief from symptoms that may interfere with normal sleep. It is helpful for muscle spasms and headaches and is used to treat nervousness, indigestion, dizziness and insomnia.

Scot's pine (*Pinus sylvestris* – Pinaceae)
The needles and young buds are used for the relief of bronchitis, sinusitis and upper respiratory catarrh. The twigs which have been previously soaked in water are added to bath water to ease fatigue and sleeplessness.

Scullcap (*Scutellaria lateriflora* – Labiatae)
Scullcap is thought to relax nervous tension and counteract sleeplessness and was entered into the US Pharmacopoeia in 1863 as a tranquillizer. It is also believed to relieve pain, muscle cramps and spasms.

St John's wort (*Hypericum perforatum* – Hypericaceae)
Used as a sedative and also to treat menopausal problems, this herb has similar properties to older commercial antidepressants and takes 2–4 weeks to exert its effect.

Valerian (*Valeriana officinalis* – Valerianaceae)
The rhizomes and roots are used in infusions to reduce sleeplessness and promote refreshing sleep. Valerian is recognized as a sedative and can be found in conventional medical formularies. It is one of the few herbs that has been

watch out!

St John's wort (see right) can have side-effects such as nausea and dizziness, and may also react with drugs. Consult your doctor before taking it.

tested using recognized scientific techniques, research having shown improved sleep after taking valerian. In one study, interestingly, smokers were found to have particular benefit. Herbalists' claims have thus been ratified in subjective ratings and clinical laboratory studies. Although the effects of valerian shown up on EEG are not those of a conventional hypnotic, they are of sufficient interest to do further work. What evidence there is supports herbalists' recommendations that it be used for nervousness, anxiety, headache, intestinal cramps and insomnia.

Wild lettuce (*Lactuca virosa* – Asteraceae)
The tinctures and infusions of the dried leaves of wild lettuce are used to treat insomnia, restlessness and over-excitability in children, as well as adults. Historically this herb has been useful as an aid in sleep disorders since Roman times. It has also been used to relieve pain by relaxing the nerves and nerve centres. Wild lettuce is thought to promote relief from symptoms that may interfere with normal sleep. Lettuce is 95 per cent water but does contain significant quantities of beta-carotene, calcium, iron, potassium, folic acid and vitamin C, all important for promoting good health and therefore sleep.

Homeopathy

Homeopathy is a complete system of complementary medicine based on the idea that a substance that produces a set of symptoms comparable to those present in a disorder can be used to treat the disorder. In other words, like treats like. Once a compound is found, it is greatly diluted (the dilution is substantial, to the extent that the resulting dose is so minimal that by conventional standards it could not possibly be effective). The symptom complex includes indices of mental, emotional and physical

Must Know
Homeopathy
Useful homeopathic remedies for anxiety are: aconite, gelsemium and arsenicum album.

states and the remedies are prepared from extracts of plants, minerals, animal and human secretions and tissues. Homeopathic practice is highly tuned to the individual and therefore general advice is shunned. There is disputed clinical evidence that it can be beneficial.

Hydrotherapy

Hydrotherapy, or water therapy, is claimed to stimulate blood circulation, draw out heat and provide support while exercising. Its main use is in muscle, soft tissue and joint injuries, but it is also occasionally used for insomnia, the rationale being that increased blood circulation eliminates toxins that may impair sleep.

Hypnotherapy

Hypnotism in some form or another has existed for thousands of years. Ancient Egyptians and Greeks are said to have used healing trances, while African and American tribal cultures have used drumming and dancing for hypnotic effects. Putting a patient into a trance to implant suggestions for self-cure has been used by the healing professions since the 18th century (as originated by Franz Anton Mesmer). The mechanisms are not clear but it has been found useful for giving up smoking and dealing with other substance abuse. Direct effects on sleepless-ness are not proven, but if hypnotherapy can be used as an aid to anxiety reduction then some benefits may accrue.

Isocones

Isocones are rubber cones that can be strapped on to the wrists to provide stimulation of the classical acupuncture points. Clinical studies show some benefit.

Massage

Massage is one of the most popular of all relaxation therapies. It can take many forms, from simple massage for relaxation to massage incorporating aromatherapy (see page 78) or other healing therapies such as reiki and shiatsu (see overleaf).

Naturopathy

Naturopathy is a natural approach to health and healing that recognizes the integrity of the whole person. Naturopathic medicine emphasizes the treatment of disease through the stimulation, enhancement and support of the intrinsic healing capacity of the person. It is personalized so that methods of treatments are, arguably, chosen to work with the patient's vital force and support the natural healing process. The practice of naturopathic medicine is based on six underlying principles of healing: (1) the healing power of nature; (2) identification and treatment of the cause of the problem; (3) not harming the person; (4) treating the whole person; (5) the physician acting as the patient's teacher; and (6) prevention. Naturopaths use nutrition, plant substances and homeopathy, as well as physical and psychological techniques and Oriental medicine.

Polarity therapy

Polarity therapy, developed by Randolph Stone (1890-1982), asserts that energy fields and currents exist everywhere in nature, and that the flow and balance of this energy in the human body provides the underlying foundation of health. The word 'polarity' describes the energy's qualities of attraction and repulsion, the funda-mental characteristics of all energy movement. In polarity bodywork, a variety of contacts and manipulations are used to stimulate and balance the body's electromagnetic fields. The

must know
Massage
As the process of going to sleep during the night involves the brain actively directing a reduction in body temperature (see page 43), any of the alternative therapies that might promote this are likely to help. Massage, for example can help improve circulation, particularly to the hands, face and feet, where temperature loss seems to be most critical. A massage prior to going to bed, or in bed, can therefore not only ease any residual aches and pains caused by injury or being over-tense during the day, but can also facilitate sleep by improving blood-flow.

practitioner may help to process feelings and develop strategies for resolving issues causing tension. Polarity has four inter-related therapeutic methods: bodywork (the practitioner's hands assist the flow of healing energy in the client's body); diet; exercise; and self-awareness (learning to understand the sources of tension).

Reflexology (also known as zone therapy)

Reflexologists believe that the body is divided up into ten zones linked to areas of the soles of the feet. Massaging the relevant area of the foot is believed to affect the corresponding part of the body. No scientific rationale exists for this treatment but it is believed to be useful for treating ailments such as back pain.

Reiki

Reiki is a hands-on healing art developed in the early 1900s by Mikao Usui. It is good for reducing and relieving emotional symptoms, such as anxiety and depression.

must know
Reiki
• Always make sure you see a qualified reiki master.
• Reiki can be self-administered.

Shiatsu

Shiatsu is a pressure-point massage technique developed in Japan. Finger pressure is applied to specific points on the body to stimulate 'meridians' through which life energy flows. It works on the same principle as acupuncture (see page 78).

Tibetan medicine

Like Indian and Chinese medicine, Tibetan medicine is a complex but remarkably coherent body of work that, despite its ancient origins, seems to provide some answers to modern health problems, such as poor sleep. According to Tibetan medicine, a doctor's compassion is an important component for the curing of serious illness. It is similar to Indian Ayurvedic medicine as it teaches that a lack of balance between three body juices, 'wind', 'bile' and 'phlegm', leads to various disorders. In Greek medicine, these 'juices' are more than the physical equivalents of wind (breath), bile (from the gall bladder) and phlegm (bronchial mucus) they have both a mental and a spiritual element. Therefore to distinguish them from other medicines they are called: *rlung* (wind), *mkhrispa* (bile) and *badkan* (phlegm).

Insomnia is thought to be caused by disturbances to *rlung*. Treatment involves a combination of therapies. **Diet:** avoid coffee and raw foods; also avoid hot pepper, chilli and too many sweet foods. Spices and herbs recommended to promote sleep are: nutmeg, sesame, cinnamon, cumin, garlic and onions. A glass of red wine is suggested both at lunch time and an evening meal. **Lifestyle:** work should not be taken home. Listen to harmonious and calming music. Eat early in the evening, and avoid exasperating conversations while eating. A massage oil based on nutmeg and butter is also recommended. Incense therapy includes a *rlung-poe* incense stick.

Fatigue is considered to be an imbalance of *rlung* and *badkan*. Sufferers are often thought to experience cold hands and feet, poor digestion, problems of feeling heavy and weak, and difficulties with breathing. **Diet:** avoid garlic, onions and milk products in the morning, and do not eat too much at once. Have five small meals a day. Fat and salt intake should be reduced. Drink plenty of boiled water and eat warming spices such as ginger. A vegetarian diet is optimal, although fish is allowed. **Lifestyle:** avoid working at night and take naps during the day. Plan specific breaks in your day for general relaxation and meditation.

want to know more?
Take it to the next level...
- Environment 38
- Good 'sleep' foods 34
- Knowing yourself 112
- Treatments for sleep disorders 172

Other sources
- Find out more about beds at the Sleep Council. They are sponsored by bed and mattress manufacturers, but it is a useful site nonetheless: www.sleepcouncil.com
- Many alternative therapies are still considered controversial. Bandolier reviews the available evidence: www.jr2.ox.ac.uk/bandolier/booth/booths/altmed.html. To read about more extravagent claims, see: www.quackwatch.org
- For information on practising yoga, see: www.bwy.org.uk

5 Taking control

Now that you know about the factors that can affect sleep, the time has come to look at your own situation more closely. Do you feel that you are getting enough sleep? If not, why not? And how can you know how much sleep is right for *you*? Filled with self-help charts, practical tips and suggestions, this chapter will help you to find the answers and enable you to take control.

Understanding your needs

Studies show that one in four of us feels we don't get enough sleep. But how much is enough? There is evidence to suggest that the number of hours you sleep may not be as important as you think, and that the real clue to a good night's sleep lies in identifying your own individual needs.

did you know?
There is evidence to suggest that hereditary and learned factors (the sleeping habits your family instilled in you as a baby) will contribute to your sleeping habits as an adult.

How much is enough?

Most people are used to thinking of sleep sufficiency in terms of the number of hours slept. Traditional sleep dogma suggests that 'eight hours a night' is the norm, and many people think that anything less than this is abnormal.

But the truth is that there is no such thing as an ideal amount, because everyone is different and has varying needs, depending on their age, circumstances and physical and psychological make-up. Just as some people are short, and others tall, some are constitutionally long sleepers and others are not. Some people can survive on four hours' sleep and wake up refreshed (Margaret Thatcher and Napoleon are two often-quoted examples of high-achieving 'four-hour-a-nighters'). Others may sleep for ten hours and wake up exhausted – an indicator that quality of sleep may be more important than quantity.

So how can you tell if you are getting enough?

If you perpetually need an alarm clock to wake you up and you are not an 'owl' (see page 114), you probably aren't getting enough sleep. Always

Work it out for yourself

To find out how many hours sleep you need, work out the average amount of time you need to sleep in order to wake up feeling well and refreshed without using an alarm clock. Then subtract this number from 24 (the number of hours in the day) and divide the result by the same number again. For example, if you know you need eight hours' sleep, this will be 24−8=16; 16÷8=2. This means that you will need one hour's sleep for every two hours awake. Similarly, if you find you need six hours a night, this will be 24−6=18; 18÷6=3, which means you will need one hour's sleep for every three hours awake.

needing to 'catch up' on your sleep is another indicator. The key here is to listen to your body. If you wake up several times in the night, and spend the next day feeling tired and sleepy, as well as miserable, you are a poor sleeper. You will know if this is the case!

Sleep debt

Sometimes the pressure of work, commuting and general lifestyle factors can put such an intolerable load on you that it can be crucial to consider how much sleep you are getting. If you find you're permanently tired, trying to catch up with your sleep or sleeping during the day, the chances are that you're incurring a sleep debt.

Sleep debts work on the principle that any lost sleep builds up into a deficit or debt that needs to be 'paid back'. If, say, you know you are a 7.5 hours sleeper and you are only getting six hours' sleep a night, then by the end of a five-day working week you will have accumulated 5 x 1.5 hours' (= 7.5 hours)

Epworth Sleepiness Scale

In contrast to just feeling tired, how likely are you to doze off or fall asleep in the following situations? (Even if you have not done some of these things recently, try to work out how they would have affected you.) Use the following scale to choose the most appropriate number for each situation:

0 = Would never doze
1 = Slight chance of dozing
2 = Moderate chance of dozing
3 = High chance of dozing

Situation	Chance of Dozing			
Sitting and reading	0	1	2	3
Watching TV	0	1	2	3
Sitting inactive in a public place (e.g. a theatre)	0	1	2	3
Being a car passenger for an hour without a break	0	1	2	3
Lying down to rest in the afternoon	0	1	2	3
Sitting and talking to someone	0	1	2	3
Sitting quietly after lunch without alcohol	0	1	2	3
In a car, while stopping for a few minutes in traffic	0	1	2	3
Total score	0	1	2	3

A score of less than 8 indicates normal sleep function:
8–10, mild sleepiness
11–15, moderate sleepiness
16–20, severe sleepiness
21–24, excessive sleepiness

If you score above 10, you should consider what is going wrong with your sleep and why you are so sleepy. If you score 16 or more, you should think about going to your doctor to discuss what might be the problem.

sleep loss or debt. One hour's lack of sleep can be recovered the following night, but if the situation persists, the sleep debt can become cumulative, so the more sleep you miss the greater the debt you will incur.

Is sleep debt your problem? And if so, what's causing it? You may need to assess your sleep needs more fully to find out. A good way to do this may be to keep a sleep diary (see overleaf).

Excessive daytime sleepiness

If you find yourself dozing through the day, it may be worth using the Epworth Sleepiness Scale (ESS) opposite to see if you have a sleep problem. Designed and validated by Dr Murray Johns of Melbourne, Australia, this scale asks you to rate the chance of your dozing during various daytime activities.

Keeping a sleep diary

Used correctly, sleep diaries can be an invaluable way of assessing your sleep needs because they provide a clear record of your lifestyle and sleeping patterns. Slow and subtle changes in your daily routines are often hard to remember, but once you write them down, you will notice tiny but highly significant things you might not otherwise have ever been aware of.

To make a sleep diary really work for you, you will need to fill it in over a period of at least two weeks when you do not have to set your alarm to be woken up. You may need to make a point of specially setting this time aside.

Two sample diaries are shown on pages 98–101: an evening and a morning one. The evening diary is used to record what you do before going to bed, while the morning diary records the sequence of events of the previous night. Feel free to adapt them as you like. Both already contain some sample questions, but do try to add anything else you feel is relevant. Keep your diary next to your bed, so that you have it to hand as soon as you wake up.

SLEEP DIARY: MORNING

Questions	Day 1	Day 2	Day 3
Date			
What time did you go to bed ?			
What time did you turn your light off (in preparation for sleep)?			
How long do you think you took to fall asleep?			
Note the times and durations of awakenings during the night. Work out the total time you spent awake			
What was the time of your final awakening?			
Work out how long you slept during the night			
Rate your sleep quality from 1 (awful) to 5 (wonderful)			
Rate how you felt when you got up on a scale of 1 (awful) to 5 (wonderful)			
Did you take anything to help you sleep during the night?			

Day 4	Day 5	Day 6	Day 7
Date			

SLEEP DIARY: EVENING

Questions	Day 1	Day 2	Day 3
Date			
Have you drunk any coffee or alcohol today? How much and when?			
When was your last meal? What did you have?			
Did you sleep during the day today? How much and when?			
How did you feel today? lethargic a little tired depressed average energetic			

As you fill in your diary, note down any changes you make in your diet or sleeping routines, and see if they make a difference. Remember, you will need to fill it in for at least 2–4 weeks to monitor yourself properly and see any new sleeping patterns emerge. Some problems can be detected over a few days; others, especially circadian rhythm disorders (see page 139), may take longer to pinpoint.

Keeping a sleep diary is never wasted. Even if your sleep problem becomes severe, a sleep professional will be able to use it to help locate the source of your difficulties.

Day 4	Day 5	Day 6	Day 7
Date			

watch out!

If you have got up in the night, be sure to make a note in your diary of why. Sometimes it is the seemingly insignificant details that may hold the key to your problems.

More ways to use your diary

Your diary is not only useful for giving you a general idea of your sleep habits. By looking at parts of it in greater detail, you can analyze your problems and tackle your sleep issues head on.

Average sleep duration

Average your total sleep time during the period of the diary (at least one week). Most young-to-middle-aged adults sleep between 5.5 and 9.5 hours. The absolute requirement varies between individuals, and on the whole is unknown. It is useful, however, to know your average sleep duration because it will not only guide you on how much sleep you need but can also be used in some treatment regimes, such as CBT (see page 172). The average sleep duration is often used as the maximum time to stay in bed when someone is relearning to sleep continuously.

How long to stay in bed?

Use a sleep diary to measure and calculate your average sleep time. If you are trying to improve your sleep duration, use this to determine how long you should stay in bed to sleep. This may initially involve some sleep restriction as you probably won't fall asleep quickly. However, within a short space of time (up to a week) you should be sleeping for this duration. Your time in bed can then be gradually increased (say 15–30 minutes each week). Approximately five hours is the minimum time to spend in bed.

Average sleep onset and awakening times

Calculate these from your diary. They provide a guide as to when to go to bed and when to get up, so as to avoid long periods of time in bed when you are not sleeping. If you note in your diary that you use your bed a lot for reading, watching television, listening to the radio, or simply lying there awake, then you need to rethink your bedtime habits. You should really restrict your time in bed for sleep (and sex if appropriate).

Getting up

If you do have problems falling asleep or waking up then you can use the average times of going to sleep and awakening as a guide as to when to go to bed and when to get up. As a rule, don't spend more than 20 minutes in bed awake. It is best to set your alarm clock for the time you usually awaken.

What time to go to bed?

If you are aiming to get to sleep quickly, take your average awakening time and subtract from this your average sleep duration. For example, if you usually wake at 5.30 a.m., and your usual sleep duration is five hours, then go to bed at 00.30 (half-past midnight).

Stimulus control

If you find that you spend a lot of time in bed awake when you hope to fall asleep then you should consider one of the behavioural techniques used to help insomniacs (see pages 172–4). A common piece of advice is that if you spend longer than 20 minutes in bed awake and cannot sleep, you should leave the bed and bedroom and not return until you feel sleepy. Opinion is divided as to whether to engage in any activity during your 'time out', but evidence does appear to indicate that the more active you are, the longer it can take to go back to sleep. So the best advice is to go and relax in another room, where you won't overstimulate the brain.

did you know?
- People who spend less than four hours in bed asleep at night are 70 per cent more likely to be obese than those who sleep 7–9 hours per night.
- Men who burn the midnight oil are more likely to become diabetic than those who don't.
- Sleeping for less than 7.5 hours increases the risk of being injured by 61 per cent.

Lifestyle

Unfortunately, we now live in a 24/7 society, which means there are times when we cannot get enough sleep. Travel schedules, shift work and family all conspire to prevent us from sleeping.

Driving

Driving is something that few of us can avoid, but is one of the biggest casualties of problem sleeping, particularly in monotonous situations such as motorway driving, where lack of concentration and vigilance can often have fatal results. Making sure you are well rested before beginning a long drive is essential, but it's also important to know what to do when you start to feel tired.

As in all aspects of sleep, two processes are at work here: (a) the pressure for sleep caused by the length of time you are awake; and (b) the pressures imposed by the biological clock 'time'. In terms of the latter, times to be most wary of are roughly between 4 a.m. and 6 a.m. in the morning, and mid-afternoon. The former period (effects of drinking, etc. aside) is associated with many road accidents, especially among young drivers. Older drivers should be particularly wary of the afternoons.

Exercise and sports

It is a commonly held view that taking more exercise improves sleep. However, although this makes perfect sense, there is, curiously, no scientific evidence to back it up. It may be that exercise has a beneficial effect on mood and general wellbeing, thus relieving anxiety and depression, which are common causes of sleep disorders. Equally, sleep and circadian rhythms (see page 14) can have an effect on certain sports, particularly

Top tips before embarking on a long drive

- Start the trip feeling well and rested.
- Avoid setting out on a long drive after having worked a full day.
- Plan the journey to include regular rest breaks, with at least 15 minutes every two hours.
- If necessary plan an overnight stop.
- Do not drive if taking medication that states on the packaging that driving or operating machinery is contraindicated, or if your doctor has told you not to drive.
- Avoid driving at times when you would normally expect to fall asleep.
- Avoid driving in the small hours (between 2 a.m. and 6 a.m.).
- Be extra careful when driving between 2 p.m. and 4 p.m., especially after eating a meal or drinking alcohol, or if you are elderly and retired.
- If you start to feel sleepy during a journey, stop somewhere safe, drink something containing caffeine and take a short nap (of about 30 minutes).

Watch out if you have any of the following symptoms

- heavy eyelids
- strained eyes and blurred vision
- an inability to keep your head up
- an inability to stop yawning
- disconnected thoughts
- total unawareness of driving the last few miles

If you do any of the following, you will be affecting other drivers too

- drive too close to the vehicle in front
- miss road signs
- unintentionally cross into other lanes or hit catseyes or speed bumps
- have problems in maintaining the speed you want

EXPERIENCE ANY OF THE ABOVE AND IT IS TIME TO GET OFF THE ROAD AND TAKE A NAP!

those that depend on muscle efficiency and joint flexibility. Performance tends to increase as body temperature rises, which may account for the fact that most records are broken in the early evening.

Sleep can also have an effect on mental performance. However, strong motivation can overcome the effects of sleepiness, and if the participants are well rested before an event, such as an exam, then even a major disruption of sleep the night before is unlikely to impair performance significantly.

The effects of long-distance travel are strongly influenced by the biological clock and if athletes are having to perform early, it is best for them to work to a 'home' rather than an 'away' time.

In the USA, researchers studied 8495 regular games in the National Basketball Association over eight seasons (1987 through to 1994) to analyze the effects of travel and rest on performance. Their conclusions were that peak performance occurred when there were three days between games. (The negative effects of little time between games may have been due to lack of time for physical recovery.) Unlike the results of earlier studies, few consistent effects in terms of distance travelled or direction of travel were found, but studies of the effects of circadian rhythms on players in some of the games on either coast in which the visiting team travelled across the country, while the home team did not travel, showed that the visiting team did better when they travelled west to east rather than east to west.

Long-distance air travel and jet lag

Ordinary long-haul commercial flying imposes various problems for travellers such as difficult timetables, getting to and from the airports, security, immigration, customs control, pressure changes and low humidity in the cabin, along with immobility, noise, vibration, radiation and – if crossing time zones – jet lag.

Unless you get the chance to travel the world by cruise-ship and other relatively slow means, you will almost certainly find yourself suffering from jet lag at some point in your life. Jet lag is caused by two factors: (a) your biological clock trying to work at a time it is not used to; and (b) the clock trying to adjust. A third major factor that causes discomfort is the stress induced by the journey itself, and its effects on sleep and the mind and body in general.

Most airlines control cabin pressure so that the maximum height experienced by the passenger is 2450m (8000ft). Even so, inside the cabin the reduced pressure effectively reduces the amount of oxygen in the blood; it also means that gases inside the body expand, which can contribute to discomfort.

Travelling across time zones

Even travelling across one or two time zones can have an effect on people who are sensitive to their biological clock time. A one-hour, one-time zone difference equates to most daylight savings adjustments. In the spring, clocks are usually moved forward one hour – so you lose an hour in bed. This is the same as travelling one time zone eastwards (e.g. travelling from London to Paris). In the winter, the clocks usually move back, so you get an extra hour in bed, and this is the same as travelling one hour westwards (e.g. Paris to London). The clock change usually occurs over a Sunday as this one-hour shift, although slight, can be enough to create problems with both going to sleep and waking up. The effects during the day are less noticeable, but hurrying to work by car because you have overslept can have disastrous consequences. In addition, mental and athletic performance, kidney function and appetite are all slightly affected.

did you know?
- Extroverts and fit and young individuals seem to cope with jet lag best.
- Night 'owls' manage better than morning 'larks'.

Travelling long distances

If you are travelling long distances, the differences will become more exaggerated. For example, travelling from London to Singapore means a long flight of around 12–12.5 hours. Singapore is east of London and is usually, depending on daylight savings, eight time zones ahead. If you catch a flight in the morning (say 11.15 a.m.) then, roughly 12.5 hours later, the plane will arrive in Singapore at 11.45 p.m. (London time), 7.45 a.m. (Singapore time). This means that the time of maximum sleepiness, and also the critical time for your bodyclock, will be around mid-day Singapore time. Your biological clock's response to ordinary daylight will be to slow down and then speed up, without really adjusting to the new zone. Mental and physical performance will also be very poor around this time.

Top tips for travelling long distances

Before the flight

- Avoid morning departures.
- Avoid 'red-eye' (overnight) flights.
- Try to reach your destination the day before your meeting so that you can aim for a whole night's sleep.
- Try to use airlines that provide flat beds so that you can stretch out as much as you can.
- Pack 'defensively': put eye-masks, ear-plugs, socks, balms, decongestants, water and moisturizers in your hand luggage.
- Wear loose-fitting clothing.
- Try to reset your bodyclock if you can – for eastbound flights, go to bed earlier and set your alarm to awaken earlier each day; for westbound flights, stay up later and get up later.
- Hope that you can get a seat away from crying infants!
- Use an airline that has pre-flight dining facilities; this usually enables you to sleep throughout the flight.

Fatigue

Fatigue is often reported after long-duration flights. However, this may in large part be due to hypoxia, or lack of oxygen, caused by cabin pressurization, and because of the disruption of circadian rhythms, irrespective of the number of time zones crossed. A study assessing the effects of hypoxia at 2450m (8000ft) and 3657m (12,000ft) showed significant effects at both altitudes.

At the 3657m (12,000ft) exposure, the effect was age-dependent, with the impact only seen in the younger subjects (23–28 years). Analysis of heart rate showed that the older subjects (29–39 years) had a greater problem than the younger subjects during the 3657m exposure. These results indicate that individual factors such as age, physical fitness and reactivity to lack of oxygen all have an impact on the body's internal clock.

Top tips for travelling long distances

During the flight
- Avoid rows near to the galley and toilet where activity, and therefore noise levels, will be greater.
- Change your watch to the destination time – it will help you adjust to the new time zone.
- Aircraft cabins are dry and everyone loses water during a flight so keep drinking water to rehydrate.
- Avoid alcohol. It may help encourage sleepiness (reduced oxygen pressure levels in cabins mean that alcohol will have a more powerful effect than usual) but it will also promote snoring and disturb sleep.
- Exercise your muscles to reduce the chances of blood clotting (try the Pilates-type movements that airlines usually describe in their in-flight magazines, or walk up and down the cabin occasionally).
- If you're going to work on the flight, do so at the beginning of the journey, then sleep (studies show it can improve memory).
- Loosen your clothing and stretch out as much as you can.

Top tips for travelling long distances (cont.)

At your destination/hotel

- Try limiting the noise in your room.
- Ask for an east- or south-facing room to get the morning sun if you are north of the equator; an east- or north-facing room if you are south of the equator.
- Make sure there are heavy curtains to block out the light (see page 39).
- Maintain your room temperature at around 18°C (65°F).
- Make sure your pillows are comfortable.
- Use a nightlight.
- Change your room straightaway if not happy!
- Put a 'Do not disturb' sign outside your room.
- Use a jet-lag calculator to work out light and dark exposure.
- Adopt local meal times and sleep-wake patterns as soon as you arrive.
- Avoid staying indoors if you are adapting or you may get sleepy.
- Get some exercise that helps loosen up the muscles and joints, thus reducing stiffness and pain. It may help reduce your appetite.

Shift work

Most shift workers have sleep of poorer quality and shorter duration than non-shift workers because of the disruption to their circadian rhythms. This can have devastating conse-quences. Evidence from the USA shows that doctors who work extended shifts of 24 hours or longer more than double their risk of being involved in a road accident on their journey home compared with those working shorter shifts. The likelihood of crashing on the way home is also greater following a night shift than after daytime shifts.

A fundamental aspect of being a successful night worker is learning how to manage your daytime sleep and fatigue at night so that you keep your sleep debt to a minimum.

Napping and 'anchor sleeps'

A nap during the night can be an essential tool for maintaining vigilance and alertness when doing shift work. The UK Royal College of Physicians recommends a 30-minute nap after every four hours worked and suggests that night-shift naps should be between 30 and 45 minutes only, as any longer than this is likely to result in the onset of deep sleep. As it is very difficult to wake up out of deep sleep and there can be considerable grogginess and performance impairment for 20–30 minutes afterwards, it may be sensible to either use an alarm clock or organize an alarm call. If a series of consecutive night shifts is scheduled, it is best to avoid prolonged sleeping during the night, rather than just napping as more sleep during the night may mean less sleep during the day.

Sleep inertia is a period of impaired performance that lasts between 5–20 minutes after awakening and which may be a problem after a nap. US Air Force crews are prohibited from napping when on immediate alert or standby because of this.

If you are engaged in an endurance activity that could take several days or more, consider having 'anchor sleeps'. 'Anchor sleeps' were first investigated in the early 1980s, when an eight-hour sleep period was divided into two four-hour periods and one of those four-hour periods was kept to the same time every day. If the anchor sleep was maintained, the circadian rhythms were found to stabilize themselves. For endurance individuals (and shift workers and parents of young children), this can be helpful, as they can choose an anchor sleep period that is more or less constant.

did you know?

British yachtswoman Ellen MacArthur sailed into the record books after completing the Vendée Globe solo round-the-world race in 2001. She became the fastest woman sailor around the globe. Ellen managed to survive on about five-and-a-half hours' sleep a day, but never in one chunk. Instead, she divided it into short naps. This enabled her to sleep as efficiently as possible, to make the most of her time in bed and maximize her active sailing time. Her average time asleep was just 36 minutes and during her 94-day voyage Ellen had 891 naps.

Knowing yourself

Keeping a sleep diary is an excellent way of getting to the root of your sleeping difficulties. But even this may not be enough on its own. To really understand what's going on, you may need to look further into the way you lead your life. Use the self-help tables on these pages to help you.

must know

Sleep assessment
The tables on these pages may not in themselves provide a definitive assessment of your sleeping problems, but they may offer clues. When in doubt, always seek a professional opinion.

Using the self-help tables

The self-help tables that follow are designed to help you pinpoint the cause of your sleeping problems by closely exploring your personality and lifestyle. Look at the questions in the left-hand column of each table, then state whether you agree or disagree by ticking the 'yes' or 'no' boxes in the right-hand column. (There is no such thing as a 'don't know' here, so if you're not sure of the answer, try to think of your tendencies on balance.) Some of the questions may be difficult, but try to answer as honestly as you can. To find out how you score in each, see page 117.

1 Lifestyle

Questions	Yes	No
Are you overweight?	☐	☐
Do you avoid exercise of any sort?	☐	☐
Do you abuse your sleep?	☐	☐
Do you have problems staying awake during the day?	☐	☐
Do you smoke?	☐	☐
Do you work night shifts?	☐	☐
Do you eat all the 'wrong' things?	☐	☐

2 Eating

Questions	Yes	No
Do you eat fish?	☐	☐
Do you eat at least five portions of fruit and vegetables a day?	☐	☐
Do you eat wholegrain foods (bread, rice or pasta) every week?	☐	☐
Do you drink alcohol in moderation regularly?	☐	☐
Do you take a multivitamin tablet with iron and folate daily?	☐	☐
Do you drink up to four cups of coffee a day?	☐	☐
Would you say that you had a balanced diet?	☐	☐
Do you avoid buying foods with a high salt or fat content?	☐	☐
Do you avoid snacking late at night?	☐	☐
Do you follow the 20/80 rule (see page 117)?	☐	☐
Do you avoid eating your dinner late at night, just before you go to bed?	☐	☐

3 Sleep worries

Questions	Yes	No
Do you ever lie in bed and worry about your inabiliy to get to sleep?	☐	☐
Do you worry about work the next day when you are trying to sleep?	☐	☐
Does your mind race when you go to bed or when you wake in the night?	☐	☐
In bed, do you plan what you are going to do the next day?	☐	☐
Does it take a long time for your brain to 'unwind' after a stressful day?	☐	☐
Do you find yourself worrying for everyone else?	☐	☐
Do you panic if you think you have woken up too early?	☐	☐
Do you worry about how bad you are at sleeping?	☐	☐
Do you keep checking the time when you are trying to get to sleep?	☐	☐
Do you often wonder how long you have been awake for?	☐	☐
Do you find it difficult to find a comfortable sleeping position?	☐	☐

4 Difficulty getting to sleep

Questions	Yes	No
Do you have to try hard to go to sleep?	☐	☐
Do you lie in bed thinking about how long you have been awake?	☐	☐
Do you get annoyed that you cannot go to sleep?	☐	☐
Do you notice any breathing or twitching as you try to sleep?	☐	☐
Do you become aware of how hot or cold you are feeling?	☐	☐
Do you find it difficult to control what you are thinking about?	☐	☐
Do you put off going to bed because you find it difficult to sleep?	☐	☐
Do you feel that you should be able to control your sleep?	☐	☐

5 Learned sleeplessness

Questions	Yes	No
Do you engage in activities other than sleep and sex in your bedroom?	☐	☐
Do you often find that you sleep better when you are not in your own bed?	☐	☐
Does your mind start to work overtime once you go to bed?	☐	☐
If you awaken during the night, do you remain in bed?	☐	☐
Do you go to bed when you are still feeling wide awake?	☐	☐

6 Larks and owls

Questions	Yes	No
Do you find that you always have to go to bed earlier than everyone else?	☐	☐
If you are going to fall asleep in company, is it always in the evening?	☐	☐
Do you awaken early?	☐	☐
Do you find that you prefer to get to bed much later than everyone else?	☐	☐
Do you find it difficult to fall asleep in the evening?	☐	☐
Are you at your worst first thing in the morning?	☐	☐

7 Restless legs

Questions	Yes	No
Do you get uncomfortable with unpleasant sensations running up and down your legs when you are trying to get to sleep?	☐	☐
Do you sometimes get the urge to move your legs when you are trying to go to sleep?	☐	☐
If you get unpleasant sensations in your legs, are they relieved when you move about?	☐	☐
Do unpleasant sensations in your legs get progressively more disturbing over the course of the night?	☐	☐

8 Sleeping pills

Questions	Yes	No
Do you take prescribed sleeping pills or tranquillizers?	☐	☐
Do you find that you have to take more and more sleeping pills for them to work?	☐	☐
Do you go to different chemists to get your sleep 'aids'?	☐	☐

9 Medicines and recreational drugs

Questions	Yes	No
Are you taking any prescribed medicine for a mental problem (such as depression, obsessive-compulsive disorder, mania or ADHD)?	☐	☐
Are you taking any prescribed medication?	☐	☐
Do you take recreational drugs regularly?	☐	☐
Do you have to take drugs to function properly?	☐	☐

10 Anxiety and depression

Questions	Yes	No
Do you often get 'butterflies' in your stomach?	☐	☐
Would you consider yourself an anxious person?	☐	☐
Do you often find that your heart is racing, your mouth is dry and that you are sweating excessively?	☐	☐
Do you often suffer from diarrhoea?	☐	☐
Are your muscles often tense?	☐	☐
Are you eating less well than you used to?	☐	☐
Are you depressed a lot of the time?	☐	☐
Do you enjoy life less than you used to?	☐	☐
Do you consider yourself to be a failure?	☐	☐
Does the future seem bleak to you?	☐	☐
Do you find that you cannot concentrate on anything?	☐	☐

11 Heavy drinking

Questions	Yes	No
Have you ever thought you should cut down on your drinking?	☐	☐
Has anyone ever told you that you should cut down on your drinking?	☐	☐
Have you ever felt bad the next day about something you did or said when you were drinking?	☐	☐
Have you ever felt the need for an alcoholic drink in the morning to get yourself going?	☐	☐
Do you drink alcohol to get yourself to sleep?	☐	☐

12 Enough sleep

Questions	Yes	No
Do you need to catch up on all your lost sleep?	☐	☐
Does sleep get deeper through the night?	☐	☐
Do you think you would look better if you got more sleep?	☐	☐
Do you need eight hours' sleep to function well?	☐	☐

Conclusions

Unless otherwise stated, if you have answered 'yes' to three or more of the questions in any of these self-help tables (with the exclusion of Table 2), you should reconsider your answers and ask yourself how long you have been behaving or feeling the way you do. Then try to follow the advice given below.

1. Lifestyle

If you answered 'yes' to all these questions then you are probably in serious trouble with regards to your health – either now or in the immediate future. It is time to change.

2. Eating

The majority of questions in this section should have been answered in the affirmative. The 20/80 rule for those who do not know it states that you can be bad 20 per cent of the time, but you must try to be good for the remaining 80 per cent. The answer to the question on coffee may also surprise you. It is not necessary to completely give up drinks containing caffeine. Just try to avoid them several hours before bed. It is possible to be exquisitely sensitive to caffeine but this is rare. Up to four cups of coffee a day have also been associated with reduced levels of colon cancer.

3. Sleep worries

Worries should be left out of the bedroom (see page 173) and you should try to adopt a wind-down routine for mind and body, so that you are ready for sleep once you go to bed. If worries start to enter your head once you are in bed, either write them down or use visualization (see page 74) or thought reduction (see page 71) to banish them.

4. Difficulty getting to sleep

Sleep is to do with letting go of wakefulness; making the decision to release yourself. 'Trying' to sleep is an active idea and will not allow sleep to come any quicker. In fact, it is unlikely to come at all. Thinking about what is going on in your own mind prior to sleep and paying too much attention to what the body is doing as you go to sleep is almost certain to lead to problems in getting to sleep (see page 71).

5. Learned sleeplessness
You may have learned to remain awake in bed as opposed to sleeping, particularly if there are no medical disorders or history that can explain your wakefulness (see page 172).

6. Larks and owls
If you answered 'yes' either to the first three questions or the last three questions then you may be suffering from a biological clock problem – go to the circadian rhythm sections in this book (see pages 14–17).

watch out!

Do not stop taking prescribed medicines or try to adjust the dosing and timing yourself – go to your GP or specialist and discuss your issue. You may be having problems with side-effects and if you intend to travel abroad, you may not have access to the advice or services available to you at home. Whatever the problem is, discuss it with a professional.

7. Restless legs
Answering 'yes' to all these questions suggests that you may have restless legs and possibly PLMD (see page 150).

8. Sleeping pills
While sleeping pills should help with difficulties sleeping, they can also be the cause of problems if taken long term. See pages 175–7 to learn more.

9. Medicines and recreational drugs
When taking prescribed medicines, it is important to be aware of any side-effects as these could disrupt your sleep. Clearly the advice for abuse of recreational drugs is to control your intake. In either case, if you are at all worried or concerned, or need help, visit your GP.

10. Anxiety and depression

If you have previously been treated for anxiety and/or depression then you should consider following any advice or treatment that has been effective before. Additionally for anxiety, you might try the breathing and relaxation exercises and alternative therapies on pages 68–91. If your current mood is poor then consider seeking further help. Depression is often associated with early-morning awakening.

11. Heavy drinking

Be wary if you have answered 'yes' to all these question – this may indicate that you are on the road towards alcoholism. Large doses of alcohol can impair sleep.

12. Enough sleep

The answers to all these questions should be 'no.' If not, go back and reread chapters 1 and 2.

want to know more?

Taking it to the next level...

- Alternative therapies 78
- Breathing and relaxation techniques 68
- Circadian rhythm disorders 139
- Clocks, cycles and rhythms 14
- Insomnia 127
- Lifestyle 36
- Sleep-related breathing disorders 132

Other sources

- To read up on tips for a healthier lifestyle, see: www.ebandolier.com
- For advice on dealing with shift work and jet lag, see: www.circadian.com, www.ba.com/arriveready, www.goodsleep.com

6 Sleep disorders

Some sleeping problems are medically classified as sleeping disorders. Many are serious, and most will need specialist care. This chapter looks at different categories of clinical sleep disorder and at other medical conditions that can disrupt sleep.

Sleep disorders

As sleep research turned into 'sleep medicine', the need arose to classify sleep disorders so as to improve treatment. The main system used is the International Classification of Sleep Disorders. The chart below is loosely based on this Classification.

INSOMNIA
- Adjustment insomnia
- Psychophysiological insomnia
- Paradoxical insomnia
- Idiopathic insomnia
- Insomnia due to mental disorder
- Inadequate sleep hygiene
- Behavioural insomnia of childhood
- Insomnia due to drug or substance (alcohol)
- Insomnia due to medical condition
- Insomnia not due to substance or known physiological condition, unspecified
- Physiological (organic) insomnia, unspecified

SLEEP-RELATED BREATHING DISORDERS

Central Sleep Apnoea syndromes
- Primary central sleep apnoea
- Central sleep apnoea due to cheyne strokes breathing pattern
- Central sleep apnoea due to high-altitude periodic breathing
- Central sleep apnoea due to medical condition not cheyne strokes

Obstructive Sleep Apnoea syndromes
- Obstructive sleep apnoea, adult, paediatric
- Sleep-related hypoventilation/hypoxaemic syndromes
- Sleep-related non-obstructive alveolar hypoventilation, idiopathic

- Congenital central alveolar hypoventilation syndrome
- Lower-airways obstruction
- Neuromuscular and chest wall disorders
- Pulmonary parenchyma or vascular pathology
- Sleep apnoea/sleep-related breathing disorder, unspecified

HYPERSOMNIAS OF CENTRAL ORIGIN NOT DUE TO CIRCADIAN RHYTHM SLEEP DISORDER, SLEEP-RELATED BREATHING DISORDER, OR OTHER CAUSES OF DISTURBED NOCTURNAL SLEEP

- Narcolepsy with Cataplexy
- Narcolepsy without Cataplexy
- Narcolepsy, due to medical condition
- Narcolepsy, unspecified

Recurrent hypersomnia

- Kleine-Levin syndrome
- Menstrual-related hypersomnia
- Idiopathic hypersomnia with long sleep time
- Idiopathic hypersomnia without long sleep time
- Behaviourally induced insufficient sleep syndrome
- Hypersomnia due to medical condition
- Hypersomnia due to drug or substance (alcohol)
- Hypersomnia not due to substance
- Known physiological condition
- Physiological hypersomnia, unspecified

CIRCADIAN RHYTHM SLEEP DISORDER

- Delayed sleep phase syndrome
- Advanced sleep phase syndrome
- Non-24-hour sleep–wake syndrome
- Non-entrained type (free-running)
- Jet-lag type
- Shift-work disorder

- Due to medical condition
- Due to drug or substance (alcohol)
- Other

PARASOMNIA

Disorders of arousal from non-REM sleep
- Confusional arousals
- Sleepwalking
- Sleep terrors

Parasomnias usually associated with REM sleep
- REM sleep behaviour disorder
- Recurrent isolated sleep paralysis
- Nightmare disorder

Other parasomnias
- Sleep-related dissociative disorders
- Sleep enuresis
- Sleep-related groaning (Catathrenia)
- Exploding-head syndrome
- Sleep-related hallucinations
- Sleep-related eating disorder
- Parasomnia, unspecified
- Parasomnias due to drug or substance (alcohol)
- Parasomnias due to medical condition

SLEEP-RELATED MOVEMENT DISORDERS
- Restless legs syndrome
- Periodic limb movement disorder
- Sleep-related leg cramps
- Sleep-related bruxism
- Sleep-related rhythmic movement disorder
- Sleep-related movement disorder, unspecified
- Sleep-related movement disorder due to drug or substance (alcohol)
- Sleep-related movement disorder due to medical condition

ISOLATED SYMPTOMS, APPARENTLY NORMAL VARIANTS AND UNRESOLVED ISSUES

- Long sleepers
- Short sleepers
- Snoring
- Sleep talking
- Sleep starts (hypnic jerks)
- Benign sleep myoclonus of infancy
- Hypnagogic foot tremor and alternating leg-muscle activation during sleep
- Propriospinal myoclonus at sleep onset
- Excessive fragmentary myoclonus

OTHER SLEEP DISORDERS

- Physiological sleep disorder, unspecified
- Environmental sleep disorder
- Fatal familial insomnia

COMMON CAUSES OF DAYTIME SLEEPINESS IN CHILDREN

Insufficient sleep

Behavioural

- Sleep-onset associations not learned
- Limit-setting problems
- Timing of sleep suits family but not child

Circadian rhythm sleep disorders

- Delayed sleep phase syndrome
- Sleep entrainment difficulties (in blind children and those with developmental delay)

Sleep fragmentation

- Behavioural (sleep-onset association disorder)
- Sleep-related breathing disorders (snoring, sleep apnoea)
- Parasomnias (night terrors, sleep talking, sleepwalking)
- Medical causes (asthma, eczema, epilepsy)
- Environmental causes (noise, light)

Increased need for sleep

Temporary sleepiness
- Medical illness
- Drug use (illicit and prescribed)

Recurrent sleepiness
- Depression
- Kleine–Levin syndrome (periodic hypersomnia, hyperphagia, hypersexuality and abnormal behaviours)
- Menstrual-related hypersomnia

Narcolepsy
- Excessive daytime sleepiness
- Cataplexy
- Sleep onset hallucinations
- Sleep paralysis

Parasomnias

Sleep-wake transition disorders
- Rhythmic movement disorder – repetitive movements involving large muscles usually occurring at sleep onset. Seen in up to two-thirds of children, usually boys, up to age four
- Sleep starts – normal, but sudden, brief muscle contractions when falling asleep
- Sleepwalking (called somnambulism)
- Sleep talking (called somniloquy)

Arousal disorders (usually settle with time)
- Confusional arousals (confusion after waking from sleep)
- Night terrors

Rapid eye movement (REM) sleep-related disorders
- Nightmares
- Sleep paralysis (unable to move or speak just before dropping off to sleep or on fully awakening from sleep). Most children will experience this at some stage
- REM sleep behaviour disorder, a rare disorder; child may act out dreams

Insomnia

As we have already seen in Chapter 2 (see pages 26–7), insomnia has various definitions but is generally defined as a difficulty in either falling asleep, staying asleep, or having unrefreshing sleep.

Insomnia can have a significant impact on a person's ability to function both socially and physically, affecting their quality of life as well as their ability to work.

It is not clear whether there is an underlying organic cause of insomnia. Some people feel that a low internal sleep pressure mechanism may be at work. Insomniac patients monitored on an EEG produce fewer slow waves after one night's sleep deprivation than normal controls and produce a larger number of fast brainwaves during the night than subjects without an insomnia problem.

Sleeplessness caused by a known disturbance is not insomnia, but insomnia can be a long-term consequence. Sleep disruption in hospital is regarded as the classic example of a precipitating cause of short-term insomnia, with hospital noise the most frequently cited cause, but certain patient care activities have been shown to be just as disruptive. Cardiac patients report greater sleep disturbance in hospital and in the first week after surgery than other surgical patients. Rearing young children is another classic cause of sleeplessness, but it does not necessarily lead to insomnia.

It has been noted that insomniac patients may be hyperaroused (a state of increased alertness, with accelerated heart rate and breathing), and that this hyperarousal may prevent them from falling asleep

> **must know**
>
> **Depression**
> A recent large-scale study conducted by the UK's Office of National Statistics investigated the incidence of depression and anxiety and found that the most common symptoms for more than 30 per cent of the population were sleep problems and fatigue. Around 20 per cent of these were both irritable and worried. Only 5 per cent experienced phobias, compulsions and panic.

must know

Adjustment insomnia

Also known as acute insomnia or sleeplessness, adjustment insomnia is thought to affect 15–20 per cent of people. Identifying the main causes is difficult but common ones are:
• problems with interpersonal relationships
• bereavement
• personal loss
• diagnosis of a medical condition
• occupational stress
• changes to sleep environment

and maintaining sleep. If normal sleepers and insomniacs are compared, the insomniacs are found to have symptoms such as increased tension and confusion, decreased vigour, some personality disturbance, subjective overestimates of poor sleep, increased body temperature and increased metabolic rate, some of which may be caused by the hyperarousal itself rather than sleep deprivation.

Mental overactivity, physical tension, fear, anxiety, stress and erratic sleep schedules are other examples of perpetuating factors. Patients whose sleep is disrupted often add to their health concerns by worrying about the consequences of not getting enough sleep, which in turn perpetuates the sleeplessness, leading to insomnia. This is particularly the case in psychophysiological insomnia (see overleaf).

Epidemiological surveys have found insomnia to be the most commonly reported sleep disorder in the general community. Almost 50 per cent of the general population has some symptoms, and 6–12 per cent has chronic insomnia consistent with medical diagnostic classifications. A large European study found that 58 per cent of those reporting insomnia regularly took sleep medications.

There are several different kinds of insomnia. (For a full list see page 122.) Most are treated by GPs and primary-care physicians, with the increasing involvement of psychologists and nurses. Insomnia may also be caused by mental or physical conditions, in which case it is known as 'secondary insomnia'.

Idiopathic insomnia

Also known as childhood-onset insomnia, idiopathic insomnia is a lifelong inability to get proper sleep.

This insomnia is often unremitting but the mental state of the sufferer generally remains good.

Treatment involves two simultaneous strategies: (1) all the methods described in Chapter 4 have to be employed to increase the possibility of sleep; and (2) giving low-dose, sedating antidepressants or sleeping pills (see page 175). The low-dose antidepressant is well below the dose required to act as an antidepressant, but these compounds have multiple pharmacological actions, some of which appear to be both beneficial and long-lasting.

Paradoxical insomnia

Also known as sleep-state misperception, this is a complaint of severe insomnia that, curiously, occurs without any objective evidence of any sleep disturbance having taken place. Daytime effects vary in severity but tend to be far less severe than expected, given the apparent lack of sleep. People with this disorder often report little or no sleep for one or more nights. They also describe having an intense awareness of the external environment, indicating they could be in a state of hyperarousal (see overleaf).

One feature of this disorder is a gross overestimation of the time it takes to fall asleep and an underestimate of the total sleep time. In a typical case, an overnight sleep study will show findings of fairly normal sleep duration and quality that differ greatly from the sufferer's perception of poor-quality sleep. Fewer than 5 per cent of people with insomnia symptoms have paradoxical insomnia.

must know

Paradoxical insomnia

This kind of insomnia is found in 1–2 per cent of the population but can account for 12–15 per cent of patients seen at sleep centres. The prevalence of idiopathic insomnia in the general population is probably less than 1 per cent whereas in sleep centres it is around 10 per cent. The general prevelance of paradoxical insomnia is also unknown but accounts for 5 per cent of patients at sleep clinics.

Psychophysiological insomnia

This is a form of insomnia that is associated with excessive worrying, often specifically about not being able to sleep. The condition may begin suddenly following a stressful event, such as a bereavement or even a stay in hospital, and can develop slowly over many years. It usually involves a period of disturbed sleep and eventually results in a more enduring insomnia. People with this type of sleep disorder often worry a great deal about their insomnia, and as a result, they learn to become tense and anxious as bedtime approaches.

The combination of learned sleep-preventing associations, and worries, coupled with the increase in bodily and mental tension feed into each other to make the insomnia worse. Even a simple bedtime routine may be a cue that causes tension to worsen. Often people suffering from this type of insomnia sleep better when they are not in their own bed. Many insomniacs will report that their sleep was poor anyway, even before the development of the really profound insomnia.

Individuals with psychophysiological insomnia suffer from decreased feelings of wellbeing. Impaired sleep can lead to problems with concentration and attention, poor energy and mood. Despite all of these daytime symptoms, sufferers still find it difficult to sleep during the day. It is common for those who suffer from insomnia to become fixated on their inability to sleep, and thinking about it makes sleep even harder to achieve as the mind works overtime.

Hyperarousal is a key feature of this type of insomnia (see opposite). Rapidly becoming the most accepted and successful treatment for psychophysiological insomnia is Cognitive Behavioural Therapy (CBT, see page 172).

must know

Can't sleep?

In a recent study, chronic insomniacs who misperceive their sleep (that is, have more sleep than they actually think they get), were given actigraphs to measure their sleep objectively. Their sleep subsequently improved when they were shown how much they were actually getting.

Hyperarousal in psychophysiological insomnia

The typical concerns a hyperaroused insomniac might have, together with statements they may agree with:

Beliefs about insomnia

Short-term negative consequences
- I need eight hours' sleep to feel refreshed and function well during the day.
- When I don't get the proper amount of sleep on a given night, I need to catch up the next day by napping or over the next night by sleeping longer.

Long-term negative consequences
- I am concerned that chronic insomnia may have serious consequences on my physical health.
- I am worried that I may lose control over my ability to sleep.

The need for control over insomnia
- When I have trouble getting to sleep, I should stay in bed and try harder.

Attributions

Restlessness/agitation
- I can't get into a comfortable position in bed.
- I can't get my sleep pattern into a proper routine.

Mental overactivity
- My mind keeps turning things over.
- I take a long time to unwind mentally.

Consequences of insomnia
- I spend time reading/watching TV in bed when I should be sleeping.
- I worry that I won't cope tomorrow if I don't sleep well.

Lack of sleep readiness
- I don't feel tired enough at bedtime.
- A delay and advance of sleep by 2–4 hours will lead to increased levels of fatigue, poorer mood and performance.

Sleep-related breathing disorders

These are a group of disorders that affect breathing during sleep and are generally treated in sleep disorder centres. See Useful addresses on pages 187–88 for more information.

They are characterized by disruptions of normal breathing patterns that only occur during sleep. The most common sleep-related breathing disorders are snoring and sleep apnoea, of which the most common type is Obstructive Sleep Apnoea (OSA). For a full list of sleep-related breathing disorders, see pages 123–6.

Central sleep apnoea

A form of sleep apnoea involving the central mechanisms that control breathing (see overleaf).

Obstructive Sleep Apnoea (OSA)

The most common sleep-related breathing disorder, or sleep apnoea, OSA is caused by the periodic reduction (hypopnoea) or stopping (apnoea) of breathing due to narrowing or occlusion of the upper airway during sleep. The narrowing of the airways can be caused either by an anatomical deformity (inherited or caused by injury or disease), reduced muscle tone or too much fat in the neck. People who have sleep apnoea can stop breathing for 10–30 seconds at a time while they are sleeping; and this can happen up to 400 times a night!

OSA is likely to be diagnosed if you have repeated episodes of upper-airway obstruction during sleep, usually associated with a reduction in blood oxygen

must know

Obstructive Sleep Apnoea (OSA)
OSA is linked to:
- premature death
- hypertension
- heart disease
- stroke
- road accidents

saturation. It can be associated with a characteristic snoring pattern of loud snores or brief gasps alternating with episodes of silence that usually last 20–30 seconds. The loud snoring may have been present for many years and can be so loud that it disturbs the sleep of partners. If you have OSA you will occasionally hear the snoring, but won't normally be aware of its intensity.

Excessive sleepiness is often the main complaint with this condition. The drowsiness is most obvious when you are in a relaxing situation such as sitting or watching television, but it also occurs in group meetings, or – in severe cases – while you are talking to someone. Naps tend to be unrefreshing and may be accompanied by a dull headache upon awakening. The daytime sleepiness can be incapacitating, resulting in accidents, self-injury and marital and family problems.

The first stage in any treatment of OSA will be to look at your lifestyle, and there may be initial recommendations to lose weight, reduce or cut out alcohol and tobacco, and avoid sleep deprivation and sleeping pills. Minor adjustments to sleeping positions (such as sleeping on the side rather than the back) may also help. If the OSA does not abate, further treatment will depend on the severity of the condition. In mild cases, an REM sleep suppressant may be prescribed; in moderate cases, removal of the tonsils and/or adenoids may he helpful; alternatively, a Continuous Positive Airway Pressure (CPAP) device (see page 183) may be recommended. If these do not work, then surgery may be an option.

watch out!

Who is most at risk?
Middle-aged, overweight men, who snore, have a collar size greater than 16 and have problems with being sleepy and staying awake during the day (e.g. at meetings, watching TV, working, driving, reading) are most likely to have OSA.

Snoring

- There is a ten-fold increase in the risk of stroke among habitual snorers.
- Snoring is a risk factor for stroke during sleep or during the first 30 minutes after waking.

Sleep apnoea

Sleep apnoea is a general term that means not breathing during sleep and is the most common form of sleep-related breathing disorder. There are several different types of sleep apnoea, the most common of which are Obstructive Sleep Apnoeas. OSAs involve a physical obstruction to the upper airways, as opposed to central sleep apnoeas, which involve a failure in breathing control. Most apnoeas are strongly related to snoring.

Snoring

Snoring is a sleep-related breathing problem. Clinically it is defined as loud upper-airway breathing caused by vibrations of the tissues behind the mouth and nose. Practically it can be both quite deafening and damaging: it eventually affects muscle tone in the neck muscles so that they collapse and obstruct breathing.

During waking, normally the muscles in the neck act against gravity and prevent the airways from collapsing. With every intake of breath there is a possibility that the airways may be sucked closed, so the neck muscles automatically tense to prevent this from happening. But when you lie on your back, as when asleep, the effects of gravity increase. This combined with the general decline of muscle tone in sleep, increases the chance of the airways being sucked closed, or partially closed. A partial closure is associated with turbulent airflow that produces noise, and this is the snore. Snoring is most commonly observed during deep sleep. It is associated with being male and has a clear link with overweight and obesity. Alcohol, tranquillizers,

Regular didgeridoo playing is an effective treatment for moderate OSA. It has also been claimed that regular singing exercise can also help. These treatments may help because they increase the muscle tone in the neck and may therefore prevent the weight of the neck (fat and muscle) collapsing on to the airways.

sleeping pills and smoking all exacerbate snoring. The cartilage in the nose and cavities behind it can also cause snoring.

How to stop

As snoring is both disruptive and extremely common, it has led to numerous inventions, devices and treatments to alleviate it. Despite this there is no universal cure, possibly because there are a number of different anatomical causes.

Losing weight, not sleeping on the back and limiting alcohol intake can help, as can nasal dilators, if nasal obstruction is the cause.

Despite the ambitious claims of many anti-snoring solutions, few have been found to be effective. In a recent experiment, an oral spray lubricant, a nasal strip to aid dilation of the nostrils and a head-positioning pillow were compared. The first product contained multiple vitamins (E and B_6) and oils (sunflower, olive, peppermint and sesame) and was sprayed into the back of the throat before bedtime. The lubricant was supposed to minimize the vibration of the soft palate. The head-position-ing pillow was designed to realign the head and neck to make breathing easier. After a week's testing, however, none of the three was found to be beneficial.

Non-surgical and surgical solutions

Clinically the most popular non-surgical methods of improving snoring use mandibular advancement or jaw-repositioning devices. These range from simple 'boil and bite' dentures to dentally fitted, self-adjustable devices that are all aimed at moving the jaw forwards. These can be successful, though side-

must know
Snoring and sleep apnoeas
Some tips on reducing snoring and sleep apnoeas:
- Don't drink alcohol before going to bed
- Avoid sleeping pills
- Stop smoking
- If necessary lose weight
- Try sleeping on your side
- Try elevating the bed head
- Go and see your doctor!

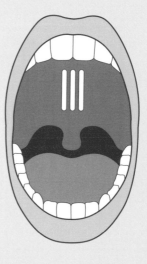

Mouth inserts

This is a new surgical procedure that treats mild sleep apnoea and reduces snoring caused by a vibrating palate. The palate is stapled with three pins.

effects may include excessive salivation, jaw-joint and dental pain and a change in the bite.

For many years the most popular surgical technique to treat snoring was laser-assisted uvulopalatopharyngoplasty (UVPP), in which the airways are surgically opened. For the right patient the success rate is high but the procedure can cause pain, and improvements often diminish over time. Alternative surgical techniques are still being explored.

Hypersomnia

This is a condition in which a person gets either too much sleep or cannot control their sleep or sleepiness. The most well-known condition is narcolepsy.

For a full list of other hypersomnias see the chart on page 123.

Narcolepsy

Narcolepsy is a chronic sleep disorder affecting one in 2000 people and is a type of hypersomnia. It affects the brain systems that control sleep, dreams and movement.

The disease is characterized by the following symptoms:

● Excessive daytime sleepiness and uncontrollable bouts of sleep.

● Insomnia.

● Dreams during wakefulness. These are generally vivid and complex, and may continue despite being interrupted by wakefulness. They can occur before the onset of sleep (hypnagogic hallucinations) or after sleep (hypnopompic hallucinations). Awareness of insects and animals are common illusions, together with feelings of flying or swooping.

● Sleep paralysis and sudden loss of muscle tone during wakefulness (cataplexy). These occur frequently and are probably a result of REM (and its associated muscle paralysis) intruding into wakefulness. Daytime cataplexy attacks usually last for a few seconds, but can be repeated for half an hour or more, sometimes even lasting an hour. They are

must know

Narcolepsy and driving
Drivers who are diagnosed with narcolepsy have a legal duty to inform the Driver and Vehicle Licensing Agency (DVLA) and their insurance companies.

usually followed by REM sleep. Cataplexy in narcolepsy is often associated with the onset of a sudden intense emotion like laughter or anger.

Narcolepsy is found in both men and women and
the first symptom is usually present before the age of
15. It can appear around the age of five, but the usual
age of onset is 20–40. In the UK there are an
estimated 20,000 narcoleptics of whom only about
20 per cent are diagnosed.

In 1999, genetic research discovered that genes
for orexin were involved in the development of
narcolepsy in animals. Subsequent measurement of
orexin levels in the cerebrospinal fluid of human
narcoleptics has confirmed the link: many narcolepsy
cases were found to be associated with either a
deficiency of orexin production or a malfunction of
the orexin receptor cell.

As well as being an inherited disorder, narcolepsy
can also be acquired. Sometimes the immune
system changes experienced during pregnancy
reveal an underlying narcolepsy, which can,
unfortunately, persist even when the pregnancy is
over. Other common causes are infections, tumours
and head trauma.

This highly disabling disorder can be treated with
stimulants (such as modafinil – see page 174),
tricyclic antidepressents (to control muscle
weakness), sleep hygiene (see page 62), and other
coping strategies. (See also Chapter 5).

must know

Narcolepsy triggers
Narcolepsy may sound
amusing but without
stimulants it can be
profoundly disabling.
Excitement, particularly
of the emotional kind,
can trigger sleep
attacks. People ringing
narcolepsy self-help
support lines that are
staffed by narcoleptics
should be aware that
the telephone ringing
can provoke a sleep
attack – so the call may
be unanswered!

Circadian rhythm sleep disorders

Studies indicate that sleep is best when it occurs at the right time, and that this is controlled by the biological clock. Unfortunately, nowadays society demands 24/7 productivity, or travelling quickly across time zones, resulting in impaired sleep. For some individuals, the biological clock itself can misbehave, making it difficult for them to work and sleep at the times society demands.

Circadian rhythm disorders are disorders of the internal bodyclock. Night-time sleep typically begins five or six hours before the body reaches its lowest temperature and finishes a few hours after this temperature is reached. For most people, this corresponds roughly to sleep onset times of between 11 p.m. and midnight, and wake-up times of between about 6 a.m. and 8 a.m. For a small percentage of the population, however, there is a misalignment between the biological clock that governs the timing of sleep and the preferred sleep–wake cycle that leads to chronic sleep disturbance. These individuals are said to have circadian rhythm sleep disorders. It is estimated that 5–10 per cent of insomniacs seeking treatment have this type of disorder.

There are several kinds of circadian rhythm disorder but they can be grouped into two general categories: (1) extrinsic (caused by some external change that has affected the natural rhythm of sleep, such as jet lag or shift work – see page 110; and (2) intrinsic (caused by the biological clock running at a different time than normal). The main symptom is

must know
Shift work
The International Classification of Sleep Disorders now recognises 'Shift Work Disorder'. It is estimated that 20 per cent of the workforce of industrialized countries has to work shifts that may include night-time or early morning work. Excessive sleepiness during a shift can be a major risk. Personal and social relationships can be adversely affected as recovery sleep often extends into the worker's free time.

usually insomnia or excessive daytime sleepiness, but unless the patient has kept a sleep diary (see page 97), it may not be immediately obvious that a circadian disorder is present.

The two most common types of circadian rhythm sleep disorder are Advanced Sleep Phase Syndrome and Delayed Sleep Phase Syndrome. Other disorders of this nature include Irregular sleep–wake pattern and Non-24-hour sleep–wake syndrome. All are treated with chronotherapy (page 180), light therapy (page 178) and melatonin (page 178).

Advanced Sleep Phase Syndrome (ASPS)

One of the two main forms of circadian rhythm disorder (the other one being Delayed Sleep Phase Syndrome). Advanced Sleep Phase Syndrome (ASPS) is marked by a chronic inability to stay awake in the evening or sleep later in the morning, or both. Many of us are natural early-morning people or 'larks', due to a slight irregularity in our internal bodyclocks, but in ASPS sufferers the distortion is so marked that bedtime can occur between 6 p.m. and 9 p.m., and waking time between 2 a.m. and 5 a.m. Although the sleep time is early, sleep itself is normal, and there is usually no major mood disturbance during waking hours, nor are normal daytime activities affected by excessive sleepiness. However, evening activities are routinely halted by the need to retire to bed much earlier than most societies regard as conventional.

One of the problems with this condition is that ASPS sufferers find it particularly difficult to adjust to new routines. Unlike people with the opposite problem, Delayed Sleep Phase Syndrome, who can simply stay in bed later in the morning to make up any sleep shortfall, ASPS sufferers can't make the same adjustments. If they stay up later in the evening, they will still get up at the same time in the morning, thereby almost certainly accumulating a sleep debt (see page 95).

Delayed Sleep Phase Syndrome (DSPS)

This is one of the two main forms of circadian rhythm disorder (the other one being ASPS). Surveys show that Delayed Sleep Phase Syndrome (DSPS) accounts for 7 per cent of all insomnia cases. Sufferers are often younger than the average insomniac patient, and many report having experienced the disorder since childhood. The average age of onset is 21 years, although on average, another six years pass before patients seek treatment.

As might be expected, on morningness/eveningness scales DSPS patients typically score as 'owls', or very-late-evening types (see also page 114).

DSPS causes progressively later and later bedtimes and later and later wake times until social constraints, such as going to school or to work, force the individual to get up. Typically, sufferers are very drowsy in the morning because they are partially sleep-deprived and because their circadian rhythm of alertness is still set for night-time sleep, then, as the day progresses they feel more and more alert. This alertness is maintained in the evenings and they often do not go to bed until after midnight, or sometimes at 2 a.m. or 3 a.m. Sufferers consistently complain of not being able to get to sleep at the proper bedtimes (but usually sleep well on holidays when they are not constrained by having set waking-up times). Absenteeism from work is a common result, and many sufferers end up doing night work because they can't hold down daytime jobs.

DSPS characteristics

Studies have shown that DSPS sufferers often show emotional characteristics such as nervousness, depression and lack of control of emotional expression. Specific personality traits include introspection, defensiveness, aspiration for

must know

Treating DSPS
DSPS is a treatable disorder but is best managed by a sleep disorders centre. The symptoms and problems are similar to those of jet lag and shift work (see page 110) except that they do not disappear by themselves. Treatment usually involves a combination of light therapy, chronotherapy and melatonin.

intellectual attainment with compulsivity, overly abstract thinking, reduced cognitive ability, neurosis, hypochondriasis and depression.

In addition, psychiatrists have observed in DSPS patients the following characteristics:

(1) an excessive defence mechanism that increases nervousness and enhances neurosis;

(2) a high level of intellectual aspiration with compulsivity that makes the patients feel self-defeated, powerless and disappointed;

(3) a tendency to egocentric emotion, inhibition and perseverance.

These characteristics may lead to withdrawal, resulting in a loss of the normal social cues that would enable a DSPS sufferer to synchronize their circadian rhythm. Thus the phase shift becomes more difficult to achieve and a vicious circle is set up.

This sleep pattern in these individuals can be quite variable. However, the majority's sleep–wake pattern drifts with their biological clocks. It is as if the biological clocks are not being entrained or synchronized by external factors. It is thought that 50 per cent of totally blind individuals have this disorder. About 70 per cent of blind individuals have problems with sleep and 40 per cent experience cyclical difficulties.

Circadian rhythm sleep disorders

Intrinsic

- Delayed sleep phase type
- Advanced sleep phase type
- Irregular sleep–wake type
- Non-entrained type (free running)

Extrinsic

- Jet lag type
- Shift work type
- Due to medical condition
- Due to drug or substance (alcohol)
- Other

Parasomnia

This is a group of sleep disorders involving either movement during sleep or seeing, hearing or feeling things that are not real.

Parasomnias include sleepwalking disorders, as well as restless legs and hallucinations around the time of going to sleep or waking up. All parasomnias are treated by neurologists and psychiatrists. For a full list see page 124.

Sleepwalking

Sleepwalking is a feature of parasomnias and is a general term used to cover disorders in which people perform some kind of activity in their sleep. The activity may consist of simple movements such as sitting up in bed and looking around, or they can be extreme such as walking or even driving a car; they can be quite benign or they can be aggressive.

The main type of sleepwalking is called somnambulism. This is most common in children, though evidence suggests that it also affects at least 1–2 per cent of adults. (The figures are unreliable because of people's reluctance to admit there are times in the night when they do things that are not under their control. Not surprisingly, some people find the complete lack of awareness of what they are doing as somnambulists very frightening.)

Somnambulism occurs during deep sleep, when the parts of the brain that decide on future planning, and whether actions are sensible or moral, are in a neutral state, but the parts of the lower brain dealing with physiological function continue to work, which explains why the walking movement can occur.

did you know?

Sleepwalkers, or somnambulists, are completely amnesic about their behaviour. Sexsomnia – having sex unknowingly during the night – is probably a specific form of somnambulism or sleepwalking.

A strong hereditary factor is believed to be involved. If both parents sleepwalk, there is a 70 per cent chance that their children will do so too.

What may set off a sleepwalking episode remains unclear, but there are clearly facilitators, or factors that increase the chances of sleepwalking occurring, and triggers during the night (see below):

did you know?

One of the first theses on sleepwalking was written in Edinburgh by Dr John Polidori (1815) who wrote the very first vampire story, pre-dating Bram Stoker's Dracula. Polidori was with Lord Byron and Mary Shelley one famous summer in Geneva, when Shelley wrote her enduring masterpiece, *Frankenstein*.

Sleepwalking facilitators
● tiredness and fatigue
● alcohol
● sleeping pills
● caffeine
● stress

Sleepwalking triggers
● sleep apnoeas
● periodic limb movements
● stress

REM Behaviour Disorder (RBD)

REM Behaviour Disorder (RBD) is a form of parasomnia involving sleepwalking. Unlike other forms of sleepwalking, which occur during deep sleep, in RBD the sleepwalking will occur during REM sleep, when the body is usually immobilized. REM Behaviour Disorder was first reported in the late 1980s and there are several types. It is diagnosed when certain symptoms are present and there is no evidence of any brain or psychiatric disorder, and no history of drug and/or alcohol abuse.

RBD sometimes begins with the onset of deep-sleep sleepwalking or sleeptalking. As the sufferer is in REM sleep, they will invariably be in a dream, although it may be a nightmare (being shot at or attacked by animals, or seeing dead people rising out of coffins, is commonly reported).

About one-third of patients with RBD will develop Parkinson's Disease (see page 162) later in life (and about 15 per cent of patients with Parkinson's will develop RBD).

REM Behaviour Disorder tends to occur in elderly men, who may not previously have had any other sleep disorder, but it can also be found in women. In one reported case study, a 35-year-old woman had waved her arms, talked and shouted in her sleep since childhood. This became a major problem when she married, and her husband eventually took to sleeping in a separate bedroom because his sleep was so disrupted by her behaviour. She became progressively depressed and eventually suicidal although there had been no psychiatric history prior to her marriage. After the diagnosis was confirmed she was treated with clonazepam which controlled her RBD and she again slept with her husband. This resolved their marital discord and her depression.

Nightmares

Nightmares are a common feature of parasomnias and there are two main types: idiopathic nightmares (where the cause is unknown) and post-traumatic nightmares (which occur as a result of a disturbing event).

Nightmares are often confused with bad dreams and night terrors, but the crucial difference is that, unlike these other two, nightmares will wake you up, leaving a detailed memory of the dream. They are highly visual, often have complicated plots, and can include several distressing and negative emotions. One piece of research noted that 62 per cent of nightmares were associated with fear or anxiety and 38 per cent with negative feelings such as anger or grief. The incidence rate of current problems with nightmares in the general population are estimated to vary between 1 and 8 per cent. More women than men report having them, but this may partly be due to the fact

must know

Personality type
Mood, anxiety and life stress are all associated with how frequently nightmares are recalled. Type A personalities (people with an insatiable appetite to succeed and compete), compared to Type B personalities (relaxed, creative and imaginative), were more likely to recall nightmares even though both personality types recall dreams equally.

that women have a better recall. However, elderly men and women have an equal prevalence of nightmares, suggesting that in women nightmares may well decline with age.

Recent research suggests that nightmares may have a genetic factor. It has also been observed that about 80-90 per cent of adults who have had nightmares in childhood report still having them 'at least sometimes', which suggests that nightmares may persist over a long time, although their frequency may change.

Sleep enuresis (bedwetting)

Sleep enuresis or bedwetting is accidental urination during sleep and is considered to be a from of parasomnia. It results from a failure to wake up when the bladder is full or from failure to prevent a bladder contraction – skills that are generally acquired with age. There is a wide range in the age when this happens. Urinating is a reflex for infants up to about 18 months. From 18 months to about three years, a child begins learning to delay urination when the bladder is full – first while awake, and then during sleep. The developmental maturity of the child will help determine the age at which this skill is gained, but most children should be able to control their bladders during sleep by the time they are about five. Thus bedwetting is not considered a sleep disorder unless it occurs at least twice a week in a person of five years of age.

Sleep hallucinations and sleep paralysis

Sleep hallucinations, along with paralysis, are common features of parasomnias and can be experienced before sleep or on awakening. Hallucinations are the most common symptom and are generally experienced as visual or auditory (see page 149), but may also include the other senses of smell, taste, movement and touch. The visions can be emotionally neutral, amusing or frightening, and can consist of small or large images that continuously or suddenly change in shape and size; sensations of actively touching or being touched; or feelings of hot and cold that sometimes move through the body. The imagery of sleep hallucinations differs from dream imagery by being shorter, more vivid and realistic, more confused and disorganized, coupled with greater awareness of the real environment.

Sleep paralysis is a temporary period of paralysis experienced before falling asleep or on REM-associated waking. Sufferers have no control over bodily movements although they are able to open their eyes and report events in their surroundings.

Vivid and terrifying sensory, motor and affective experiences often accompany sleep paralysis and there may be emotionally vivid and complex dream-like hallucinations consistent with sleep onset REM sleep. Research shows that these hallucinations fall into three major categories:

• **Incubus** (including breathing difficulties, feelings of suffocation, bodily pressure, pain and morbid thoughts of impending death).

• **Intruder** (typically including a vague sense of a threatening presence accompanied by assorted noises, footsteps, gibbering voices, humanoid apparitions and sensations of being touched or grabbed).

must know

Sleep paralysis
There is a higher prevalence of sleep paralysis among college students and those seeking treatment for anxiety disorders. Sleeping on your back increases the likelihood of sleep paralysis and the more episodes of sleep paralysis that are experienced, the more fantastic the sensations may become, and a narrative may develop.

● **Vestibular** (including sensations of acceleration, described as floating, flying and falling. Also common are out of body experiences, seeing oneself from an external view-point, and moving). See also Parasomnias.

Sleep-Related Eating Disorder (SRED)

SRED is a form of parasomnia that consists of repeated episodes of compulsive binge-eating and drinking after waking up in the night, with only a partial memory (or sometimes none at all) of what has happened. Some people are alert as they eat; others still asleep. Waking up the person during an eating episode may be very difficult and may provoke anger and resistance. There is normally no link between this condition and daytime eating disorders. In SRED, binge-eating is limited to night hours with none of the self-induced vomiting or laxative abuse that is found in anorexia nervosa or bulimia.

Most people with this disorder have an eating episode nearly every night, and some eat more than once a night. Episodes can occur at any time, and can often be very short, sometimes lasting for only ten minutes – the time taken to get from bed to the kitchen and then back to bed again. Feelings of hunger and thirst are often absent, and sufferers often eat foods they avoid during the day – high-calorie and sugary foods such as syrup generally prove the most popular. Alcoholic drinks are almost never consumed.

Careless cooking methods and sloppy food handling are a feature of this condition – people with SRED often only remember an episode on finding a very messy kitchen the following morning – and can lead to injuries such as cuts and burns, and sometimes even fires. This

Below are some of the more common visual and auditory hallucinations that have been described:

Visual

- Formless outlines (waves or clouds of colour)
- Designs (symmetrical patterns and shapes)
- Faces, figures, animals and objects
- Natural scenes (landscapes, seascapes, etc.)
- Scenes with people
- Print and writing in real or imaginary languages

Auditory

- Crashing noises
- One's name
- Doorbells and chimes ringing
- Pompous nonsense
- Quotations
- References to spoken conversations
- Meaningful responses to a thought of the moment
- Music, bangs, explosions

unusual disorder can develop suddenly or slowly. It is long-lasting and does not seem to ease up over time. It may be a factor in causing depression, which results from a sense of shame and failure to control the eating. Some sufferers avoid eating during the day and may over-exercise in an attempt to prevent obesity.

Sleep-related movement disorders

There are four main types of sleep-related movement disorder: Periodic Limb Movement Disorder, Restless Leg Syndrome, Sleep Bruxism and Sleep-Related Rhythmic Movement Disorder.

must know

Risk factor in PLMD
The largest study investigating the prevalence of PLMs (Periodic Leg Movements) found 4 per cent of 19,000 subjects suffered, with an age range of 15–100 years. Being female, drinking coffee, stress and the presence of mental disorders were all risk factors.

Periodic Limb Movement Disorder (PLMD)

PLMD is typified by periodic leg movements, sleep-related, repetitive and characteristic movements of the legs. Many sufferers may not be aware that these movements are taking place and can report non-refreshing sleep or insomnia, or daytime sleepiness. The movements will disturb sleep but not enough to bring awareness (bed partners are more likely to report the kicking and jerking). Patients with sleep apnoea (see page 134) may move their limbs periodically but these movements often disappear when the sleep apnoea is treated. Patients with PLMD may experience insomnia, fatigue and daytime sleepiness. A specialized form of actigraphy (see page 184) or sleep polysomnography is useful in confirming the diagnosis and assessing whether it is associated with any other sleep disorders.

PLMD and Restless Leg Syndrome (RLS) are both found in sleep apnoea and narcolepsy (see page 134 and 137). It is not clear why this should be but there is speculation that these disorders involve damage to roughly the same areas of the brain. Treatments include a number of different pharmacological approaches. Clonazepam or other benzodiazepines may be prescribed, or L-Dopa/carbidopaor bromocriptine, or various opioids (codeine, methadone, oxycodone and propoxyphene) may be tried before the right drug is found. More recently, pramipexole and ropinirole have been introduced for the treatment of RLS and PLMD (originally described as if they were a form of nocturnal epilepsy). Similar movements can occur in the arms but these are much rarer. Usually the toe extends and the ankle (and possibly knees and hips) flex a little. The movements are very periodic, occurring every 15–40 seconds, and can be grouped into runs of half a minute to an hour. PLMD rarely occurs in healthy children. It does, however occur in children with OSA (see page 132), juvenile fibromyalgia and ADHD (see page 153). PLMD had been found in various sleep disorders such as REM Behaviour Disorder (see page 144) and in particular in RLS.

Restless Leg Syndrome (RLS)

Restless Leg Syndrome (RLS) is a form of sleep-related movement disorder. It usually occurs at rest (in the evening and early part of the night) and involves peculiar sensations in the legs (the areas between the knees and ankles are most affected) with an often irresistible desire to move them which can often provide relief. Some patients cannot describe the sensations at all. Others will use a variety of words to describe them, generally including 'ache', 'discomfort', 'creeping', 'crawling', 'pulling', 'prickling', 'tingling' or 'itching'. These sensations are associated with a strong urge to move, and in response patients typically walk around, often rubbing, stretching and flexing their legs, tossing and turning in bed, or pacing the floor. There are also many specifically sleep-related symptoms. Studies show that RLS sufferers have a

must know

PLMD
Many psychoactive medications will increase PLMD
- clomipramine
- lithium
- fluoxetine
- venlafaxine

higher incidence (33 per cent) of sudden sleep onset than non-sufferers (20 per cent), and falling asleep while driving is reported by 15 per cent of patients. Many pregnant women (up to 15 per cent) are affected by symptoms that tend to be at their most distressing and disruptive in the third trimester of pregnancy.

RLS, like many other sleep-related disorders, comes in several forms, and the condition can be intrinsic, with no known cause, or caused by external factors such as disease. Current reports suggest a genetic factor may be involved in some forms. Mild RLS may not require medical treatment. Initial reassurance is important, and many of the symptoms may be relieved by simple lifestyle changes (see Chapter 5) and strategies such as walking and stretching, having hot or cold baths, relaxation exercises such as yoga (see page 74), massaging the affected limbs or enjoying mind-distracting activities while sitting. Secondary causes (see box opposite) of the disorder must be corrected. Dietary supplementation with iron and mineral (magnesium, potassium and calcium) supplements may be helpful.

must know

Things to avoid
Drugs that worsen RLS include:
- antidepressants
- calcium blocker drugs (for high blood pressure)
- anti-nausea medications except Domperidone
- high intake of caffeine
- some anti-allergy medications

Sleep Bruxism (tooth grinding)

A recent international study, based on 13,057 participants in Italy, Germany and the United Kingdom, has shown that the grinding or clenching of teeth during sleep on a weekly basis affects more than 8 per cent of the population and is associated with other disorders such as daytime sleepiness and anxiety. The condition is known as Sleep-Related Bruxism, and is a rhythmic activity of the jawbone muscles that causes forced contact between dental surfaces during sleep. It has been linked to headaches, joint discomfort and muscle aches, premature loss of teeth, and sleep disruption for both the person with bruxism as well as his or her bed partner.

Sleep bruxism is approximately twice as likely to occur in people with OSA (see page 132) and heavy drinkers. Increased incidence is also found in loud snorers and caffeine drinkers – and, to a lesser extent, in smokers and people with anxiety or stressful lifestyles. It is quite common among children although it usually declines with age. Only about 1 per cent of the elderly suffer from it.

In adults, bruxism may occur because of oral or dental problems, but also because of anxiety, sleep deprivation, or the effects of medicines such as L-Dopa, SSRI antidepressants and alcohol. Treatment includes improving sleep hygiene (see page 62).

Sleep-Related Rhythmic Movement Disorder

While head banging or body rocking during sleep is very common in infants and young children, less than 5 per cent of children over the age of five years old exhibit this kind of behaviour. When it does persist it has been associated with Attention Deficit/Hyperactivity Disorder (ADHD). Treatment in youngsters can be difficult but a combination of controlled sleep restriction and sleeping pills has been found to be useful. In children it occurs during light stages of sleep and it is thought to be a self-soothing behaviour. In adults, however, it has been noted in all stages of sleep.

> **must know**
>
> **RLS causes**
> Restless Leg Syndrome can be caused by the following:
> - iron deficiency anaemia
> - diabetes mellitus
> End Stage Renal Disease (ESRD)
> - folic acid deficiency
> - Parkinson's Disease
> - peripheral neuropathy fibromyalgia
> - rheumatoid arthritis
> - spinocerebellar atazia

Other conditions that affect sleep

Some forms of sleep disorder are caused by disorders and conditions that are not directly related to sleep. The new International Classification of Sleep Disorders also lists sleep disorders that are difficult to classify. Here we look at many of these other disorders as well as health conditions that are affected by sleep disorders.

must know

Alcohol and sleep

While studies show that 2–3 units of alcohol before bedtime promote sleep, this probably stops happening within a few days of continued consumption. Other studies show a strong relationship between alcohol dependence and insomnia. Alcohol should not be used to treat insomnia; alcoholics will also suffer from insomnia.

Alcoholism

The absence of deep sleep is very common in alcoholics. Chronic, long-term alcohol-use can be associated with an absence of Stage 2 sleep (see page 19) and the presence of an unusual transitional state that is similar to REM sleep and wakefulness, and is also coupled with hallucinations and dream behaviours that are acted out as in REM Sleep Behaviour Disorder (see page 144). Insomnia is one of the many reactions caused by alcohol withdrawl following habitual excessive drinking, or even after a single episode of heavy alcohol consumption. Alcoholic patients also experience lower levels of melatonin (see page 16) during the early part of the night and a delay in the onset of the nocturnal melatonin, compared with non-alcoholics.

Anxiety disorders

Many anxiety disorders are associated with insomnia. Often there are problems with falling and staying asleep. The following are the main types:

Panic disorder consists of recurrent, persistent and unexpected periods of intense fear and discomfort in the absence of any real danger. The attacks are followed by persistent concern about the implication and possibility of other attacks. The attacks have a sudden onset and peak within 10 minutes. They are accompanied by a sense of impending doom and an urge to escape. Insomnia is a common complaint in about 70 per cent of patients. Most patients will suffer from at least one nocturnal attack, usually occurring at the onset of deep sleep. Treatment consists of Cognitive Behaviour Therapy (CBT – see page 172) which deals with misappraisal of anxiety symptoms.

Post-Traumatic Stress Disorder (PTSD) – (see also page 163) develops after exposure to an event that involves intense fear, helplessness or horror. It consists of a persistent re-living of the event as well as avoidance of situations associated with the trauma. Recurring nightmares of the event are one of the hallmarks of the disorder. **Acute Stress Disorder** also follows a traumatic event but the insomnia and general disturbance is limited to one month.

Generalized Anxiety Disorder is characterized by an excessive anxiety and worry about a number of events or activities; the individual has difficulty in controlling their worries. Insomnia is common.

Chronic Fatigue Syndrome

A condition involving impairment of cognitive functions and quality of sleep, with numerous symptoms such as recurrent sore throat, muscle aches, joint pain, headache and feelings of illness after exertion. The origin is complex, currently unknown.

Dementia

A range of medical conditions that commonly cause insomnia. In fact, recent studies on sleep disturbances in

must know
Alzheimer's
Patients with Alzheimer's dementia have disturbed circadian rhythms which probably lead to increased activity in the late afternoon, early evening or, in many cases, at night. Movement and activity tend to be less during the early part of the day. There is no treatment for the disturbance to circadian rhythms, but use of bright light (see page 178) and a strict behavioural regime can help.

Alzheimer's dementia have found that the disturbances contribute to the early diagnosis of the disease. In Alzheimer's dementia the average time of night sleep is around 5.7 hours and the time spent awake is 2.7 hours. Both REM and slow wave sleep are of reduced duration with several phases of apnoea, and the circadian rhythm of melatonin is disturbed. Many dementias are progressive and unstoppable and the success of dealing with sleep problems depends on the stage the disease is at. The overall physical and mental health and life events that might contribute to the sufferer's insomnia are hard to assess. The factors that could be changed and that can improve sleep are:

- physical environment
- social life
- sleep hygiene
- physical fitness
- nutrition
- patient-carer interactions

Depression

The importance of sleep problems in depression can't be overestimated: insomnia is often the reason that makes depressed patients seek help, and relief of sleep disturbance is an important factor in most depression treatments. Research shows that depressed people have impaired sleep continuity and efficiency with increased wakefulness. Sleep-onset latency (the length of time between going to bed and falling asleep) is significantly increased and total sleep time reduced. Slow-wave sleep may be reduced and Rapid Eye Movement (REM) sleep is also affected in 40–70 per cent of depressed outpatients. Apart from the discomfort that sleep problems produce, they can also lead to exhaustion and poor functioning during the day (with a possibility of accidents) plus an associated increased risk of suicide. (See also Seasonal Affective Disorder (SAD) – see page 17.)

must know

Fibromyalgia

Fibromyalgia affects around 2 per cent of the population but 80 per cent of those afflicted are women. The disorder is not inherited but some families are more susceptible. Symptoms may start either after a feverish flu-like illness, or a work-related injury, or following a car accident whiplash-type of injury.

Fibromyalgia Syndrome

Insomnia, headache and fatigue are the most reported symptoms and are also part of the definition of this condition. The precise nature of this syndrome is still debated, with definitions changing over the years, but sleep is disturbed with a minor increase in the number of arousals. The sleep abnormality is referred to as alpha-delta sleep or alpha sleep pattern. Symptoms get worse in the winter and in cold climates. They improve in warmth, summer and after mild aerobic exercise. As similar symptoms can be produced in normal volunteers by disrupting deep sleep using noise, it has been suggested that the disorder is a deep-sleep disorder.

Restless Leg Syndrome is reported in more than 30 per cent of patients; nearly 40 per cent of young people with fibromyalgia will also have PLMD, and Obstructive Sleep Apnoea is reported in more than 40 per cent of men, but only 2 per cent of women. Fibromyalgia differs from other rheumatic conditions in that no physical reason has yet been found to account for the diffuse pain, fatigue, distress and unrefreshing sleep that is caused

must know

Epilepsy

Nocturnal frontal lobe epilepsy embraces a wide variety of sleep-related behaviours, ranging from brief sudden awakenings to prolonged periods of 'sleepwalking' behaviour which can occur several times a night. Seizures appear most frequently in the teens, and increase in frequency with age.

Epilepsy

A seizure or fit occurs when there is a sudden and excessive discharge of nerve cells. Epileptic seizures are recurrent and unprovoked attacks, which frequently occur during sleep most often as seizures starting in the frontal or temporal lobes of the brain. It is estimated that epilepsy occurs in roughly 5–10 people in every 1000 persons, athough there are large differences across ages. As there are a great many reasons why epilepsy may develop, 50–60 per cent of cases are of unknown cause. Of the 5–10 per 1000 epilepsy cases, between 10–45 per cent are thought to be sleep related, but the wide range reflects the wide variety of types. There are several types of predominantly sleep-related, nocturnal epilepsies but the best studied is Nocturnal Frontal Lobe Epilepsy. This can mimic sleepwalking, night terrors and confusional arousals (awakenings). The movements can be quite well coordinated, or simply repetitive, and may involve striking out hard and causing damage or injury. This epilepsy causes severe sleep disruption to the individual, leading to daytime fatigue and sleepiness. It can start at any age but it is most common between the ages of 10 to 16 years old. About 70 per cent of cases will respond to anti-epileptic medication.

Headaches

There is a clear association between sleep disturbances and headaches, especially with headaches that occur during the night or early morning, although which causes the other is unclear. Nevertheless, identification and treatment of sleep disorders among chronic headache sufferers is worthwhile as it is often followed by improvements in the headache. The main types of headache are as follows:

Migraine

A moderate to severe headache that often starts in the same way each time, and gets worse and worse until there is a one-sided throbbing pain that is aggravated by physical activity, and is associated with either nausea or vomiting or light or sound phobia, or some combination of all of these. Migraine headaches are often preceded by visual or auditory aura symptoms (an aura being a distinctive feeling, atmosphere, mood or sensation – a prem-onition of what might happen). Rest and sleep usually brings relief. Episodes can be frequently triggered by factors such as emotional stress, hypoglycaemia (low blood sugar), lack of sleep or

must know

Kids and migraines

Children who suffer from migraine headaches also tend to suffer from a range of sleep problems:
- bedroom resistance
- taking a long time to get to sleep
- short sleeping times
- more night-time awakening
- greater sleep anxiety
- more daytime sleepiness
- more parasomnias and disordered breathing

Heart conditions

There are several heart conditions that both affect sleep and are affected by sleep disorders:

Irregular heart beat

This can be caused by.Obstructive Sleep Apnoea (OSA). OSA sufferers may not be aware that the irregularities are occurring, so continuous 24-hour recordings may be recommended by practitioners.

High blood pressure (hypertension)

The surge of increased blood pressure upon awakening and arising may be the cause of an increased incidence of strokes (see page 163). The risk is greatest for those suffering from OSA, who can experience blood pressure increases of up to 50 per cent.

Chronic heart failure

Chronic heart failure is a common condition with a poor prognosis. It generates many debilitating symptoms for the sufferer, including sleep-disordered breathing.

excess sleep (the 'weekend migraine'), excessive sensory stim-ulation, e.g. loud noise, bright light, strong odours, heat or cold, or physical stimulation, such as sport or physical exercise. Feelings of being alert, tense, irritable, annoyed, depressed or tired and changes in the quality of sleep may occur up to two days before a migraine attack and there are reports that disrupted sleep patterns may be involved in triggering attacks. In some sufferers, over-use of medication can worsen both sleep pattern and headaches; when the medication is withdrawn, the associated sleep disturbance is alleviated along with the frequency and intensity of the headaches. Recent studies suggest that head-aches and migraine with aura may be related to extended sleep duration.

did you know?

A recent study of 740 people over a period of 12 years showed a correlation between age and an increased incidence of tension headaches. This onset of tension headaches let to:
• poor self-related health
• an inability to relax after work
• disturbed sleep

Tension-type headache

Tension-type headache is a term used by the International Headache Society to describe what previously was called tension headache, muscle contraction headache, psychogenic headache or stress headache. Chronic tension-type headache, associated with more severe pain, is often combined with medication over-use and is less influenced by the stresses of daily life, unlike tension headaches in general. Tension-type headaches are characterized by pressing pain of mild to moderate intensity on both sides of the head without the other symptoms of migraine, and may also be associated with sleep disruptors such as insomnia, hypersomnia and circadian disturbances. Poor sleep is common and sleep disturbances have been shown to play a role in chronic pain. However, no formal studies have evaluated sleep pattern and EEG activity in patients with chronic tension-type headaches.

Migraine patients have essentially normal sleep although REM sleep may be affected between attacks. Patients with tension headache, on the other hand, have reduced sleep time and sleep efficiency, may fall asleep quickly but may also have frequent awakenings, increased nocturnal movements, and marked reduction in slow-wave sleep, with little effect on REM sleep. Findings therefore suggest that patients with intermittent migraine may have minimal sleep disturbance, while more chronic headache disorders may be associated with or worsened by poor sleep. Tension headache is the most common type of headache and is regarded by most people as 'normal' compared to migraine; however, it causes more work absences than migraine.

Cluster headache

Cluster headaches are a debilitating strictly one-sided headache accompanied by a runny nose, streaming eyes or similar symptoms. They generally occur after 1–2 hours' sleep (usually at the onset of REM) and usually appear at a particular time of year, hence the term 'cluster headache'.

Cluster headaches predominantly affect men. Precipitating factors include levels of histamines, alcohol, and environmental changes, as well as alterations in levels of physical, emotional or mental activity. As cluster headaches occur mainly during sleep and as oxygen supply is effective in the treatment of acute attacks, a potential connection with sleep-disordered breathing has been suggested – the breathing disorder may not cause the headaches but it worsens the attacks. There is some evidence that Continuous Positive Airway Pressure device (see page 183) may reduce cluster headache severity. Research suggests that a lack of melatonin secretion may a relevant factor in nocturnal attacks.

Hypnic headache

The hypnic headache is a rare but recurrent, late-onset headache disorder that usually begins after the age of 60 and occurs exclusively during sleep. Headache attacks occur predominantly during night-time sleep, but may also occur during daytime naps. The mechanism is not known but some reports have suggested an association between arousals and headache episodes during REM sleep or impaired breathing. Lithium is an effective treatment in some cases, though the side-effects can be severe. Other reportedly effective drugs are flunarizine, verapamil and indomethacin.

Snoring, insomnia and headache

The relationship between disturbed sleep leading to full awakening and headaches of any type is unclear. In a US national survey of 6072 adolescents, a clear relationship between insomnia and headache was identified in less than ten of the teenagers, although an increased prevalence of insomnia, nocturnal awakening, somnambulism, enuresis and nocturnal snoring was noted in children with chronic headaches.

A large epidemiological study of 3323 males, aged 54–74 years found a positive correlation between self-reported snoring and headache. Headache was also associated with hypersomnia (see page 137), although the relationship between snoring and headache was not related to the severity of hypersomnia. In another study of 1504 males and females aged 30–60 years, only a weak link was found between snoring and headache, but sleep apnoea (see page 134) was associated with morning headache and cognitive complaints. Snoring, nightmares and headaches all showed a significant, negative correlation with age, indicating that the incidence of headaches in the elderly is related to sleep snoring and apnoea. Patients with Obstructive Sleep Apnoea (OSA – see page 132) frequently complain of excessive daytime sleepiness, chronic fatigue, snoring, morning headache and nocturnal arousals.

Myotonic dystrophy

Excessive Daytime Sleepiness (EDS) is found in one-third of patients with Myotonic Dystrophy Type 1. Sufferers report a longer sleep period, less restorative sleep, and more difficulty in falling asleep, while being alert in the morning and staying awake after meals. The severity of daytime sleepiness is related to the extent of muscular impairment.

Nocturia

Nocturia, or frequent urination at night time is a common but largely misunderstood condition in adults that can have extremely debilitating effects because of the inevitable sleep disruption involved. There are various possible causes, including bladder dysfunction, but some cases are believed to be caused by sleep apnoea.

Parkinson's Disease

Several reports have shown that most Parkinson's Disease patients suffer from sleep problems. People with this condition have reduced total sleep time compared to healthy individuals and can spend at least 30–40 per cent of the night awake. (About 80 per cent of patients report 2–5 awakenings a night.) Overall, patients and partners report problems with sleep in about 25 per cent of male Parkinson's patients and 48 per cent of female sufferers.

Parkinson's is usually progressive, so, over time, sleep problems will gradually worsen, with sufferers taking longer and longer to fall asleep and getting less sleep overall. More specifically, they will experience less deep sleep, REM sleep and considerably more wakefulness.

Vivid dreams are frequent with this condition, and can become intense, frightening and repetitive, often turning into nightmares in which the sufferers shout out and thrash around. Hallucinations, sleep talking, some sleepwalking, night terrors and panic attacks may also occur, some of which can happen in the day.

Disturbed sleep often starts early on in the disease. The causes are varied but it is likely that the underlying problem is degeneration of the sleep-promoting and sleep-maintenance centres. Sleep-disordered breathing caused by Obstructive Sleep Apnoea (OSA – see page 132) is also believed to be implicated.

Sleep disturbances in patients with Parkinson's Disease are typically under-recognized and ineffectively treated. However, effective management of sleep disruption and excessive daytime sleepiness can greatly improve the quality of life for patients with this distressing condition.

Post-Traumatic Stress Disorder (PTSD)

Studies have found that 60 per cent of Post-Traumatic Stress Disorder (PTSD) patients have nightmares that can be long-lasting. One study has found a 56 per cent incidence rate of nightmares in PTSD patients who experienced war-related traumas more than 40 years earlier.

must know

Parkinson's
Excessive daytime sleepiness can affect 20 –50 per cent of patients with Parkinson's Disease while sleep attacks or sudden bouts of sleep are infrequent. Sleepiness is often associated in the later stages of the disease and higher doses of L-Dopa and possibly the use of dopamine medicines. Patients at risk of sleep attacks have higher Epworth Sleepiness Scale (ESS) scores (see page 96) and if they are taking ergot or non-ergot dopamine medicines.

Psychoses

Insomnia is a common feature in schizophrenia and is often seen in – or may precede – exacerbations or relapses in the condition. The sleep disturbances of patients who have either never been medicated or previously treated are characterized by problems with starting and continuing sleep. More specifically slow-wave sleep is significantly reduced. Many of these problems are treated with prescription medications. The atypical antipsychotics olanzapine, risperidone and clozapine significantly increase total sleep time, while olanzapine and risperidone enhance slow-wave sleep. The typical antipsychotics haloperidol, thiothixene and flupentixol significantly reduce the time to get to sleep and increase sleep efficiency.

must know

Psychoses

Psychoses, or major mental illnesses, have long had an association with dreams or disturbed sleep (hallucinations, delusions and bizarre thought processes occur in both schizophrenia and dreaming). Treatments of Parkinson's Disease, and high-dose stimulant use in narcolepsy (see page 137) can in turn provoke psychotic symptoms.

Sleep-Related Gastro-Oesophageal Reflux

It is thought that about 10 per cent of the population suffer from heartburn, with 75 per cent experiencing symptoms 2–3 times per week. Sleep-related reflux involves bringing up stomach contents into the oesophagus during sleep. It may awaken the patient with a sour or acidic taste in the mouth, or perhaps a burning sensation in the chest. Sometimes there are no obvious symptoms but sleep is nonetheless disturbed.

Somatoform disorders

These disorders are physical symptoms that suggest a medical condition but none can be found. The symptoms are not under voluntary control but it is thought that their cause is psychological. Patients can complain of general pain, gastric disturbances, sexual problems and other neurological disturbances. Getting to and staying asleep are always an issue. Cases of disorder usually begin before the age of 30 and can be compared to hypochondriasis, in which the individual believes that they are suffering from a serious illness when none is present.

Stroke

Several recent reports have noted the prevalence of sleep apnoea (see page 134) in about 60 per cent of subjects suffering a stroke, although opinion remains divided as to whether the apnoea is an independent or a stroke-related problem. Despite big changes in blood pressure in the brain during sleep and particularly during breathing difficulties, there does not appear to be an associated increase in the occurrence of strokes during sleep, although there is an increase in the possibility of stroke in the early hours of the morning.

Obstructive Sleep Apnoea (OSA – see page 132) is common among stroke patients. But there is still some uncertainty about the link between sleep apnoeas and stroke. It is not clear, for example, whether patients with polysomnographically proven OSA are at a risk of strokes that is independent to the problem they have with their circulation. Currently, only studies based on a history of snoring support the idea that sleep-disordered breathing is an independent and significant risk factor. Doctors and sleep scientists also remain unclear as to whether the presence of sleep-disordered breathing has a negative impact on stroke outcome. Finally, there is no scientific evidence to determine whether Continuous Positive Airway Pressure (CPAP – see page 183) treatment affects the risk of either recurrence or clinical outcome, or both, in stroke patients with OSA.

want to know more?
Take it to the next level...
- Clocks, cycles and rhythms 14
- Knowing yourself 112
- REM sleep 20
- Snoring partners 42
- The brain's metronome 16
- The role of melatonin and serotonin 16–17
- Treatments for sleep disorders 172

Other sources
- For information on snoring, see www. britishsnoring.co.uk
- For information on narcolepsy, contact the Narcolepsy Association, www.narcolepsy.org.uk
- For general information, see www.sleepeducation. com. See also the American Academy of Sleep Medicine, www.aasmnet.org
- For information about insomnia, go to www.sleepspecialists. co.uk

7 Sleep medicine

For some sleeping problems, self-help
solutions may not be enough, and the time
may come to seek specialist care. This chapter
looks at the increasing role of sleep disorder
centres and some of the most popular and
proven treatments on offer.

The work of sleep clinics

Severe or protracted sleeping difficulties will require a referral to a sleep disorder centre, where your problem can be assessed more closely. But how do these sleep clinics work? This section shows you what to expect.

Types of sleep clinic

In countries where sleep disorder medicine is on the rise, two types of sleep disorder centre have evolved: (a) those that focus on snoring and sleep apnoea; and (b) those that deal with general sleep disorders. In practice, however, the prevalence of snoring and sleep apnoea – combined with the fact that most doctors in the UK who are interested in sleep are specialists in respiratory disorders – means that the former type predominates by far.

The first stage at a snoring and sleep apnoea clinic will be to assess your condition and decide whether it's serious enough to warrant treatment. One simple and common method of assessment is by using overnight oximetry (a way of measuring oxygen levels in the blood), which you can often carry out at home with a special measuring device attached to your finger.

A general sleep disorder centre will almost certainly send out a sleep diary (see page 97) and questionnaire before your appointment. What happens next will depend on what the sleep specialists decide. Depending on your condition, you may again have to undergo some kind of measurement procedure, probably carried out at home. If your problem is believed to be biological-clock-related, for example, you might be sent home with an actigraph (a wristwatch-shaped device that measures the activity of the sleep and wakefulness centres in the brain (see page 184).

Overnight monitoring

The most notable feature of most sleep disorder centres is the bedside wiring that is used for over-night monitoring. The monitoring involves gluing several tiny electrodes to the scalp and face to measure brainwaves (on the EEG), eye movement and chin muscle tone. (The glue can be dissolved with acetone or another solvent the following morning.) Since muscle tone and eye movements also differ between wakefulness and sleep, these too are measured, using electro-oculography (EOG) and electromyography (EMG). There is no need to be shaved (monitoring can, in fact, be slightly more difficult on bald heads as the electrodes tend to skid around when you are trying to apply them).

The electrodes attached to the scalp will provide enough information to identify the main stages of sleep, but, since irregularities of breathing and oxygen levels in the blood can also disturb sleep, these will need to be measured too. This will involve attaching sensors to the nose (for air-flow) and fingers (for blood oxygen levels), and attaching chest straps for breathing movements. Further electrodes may also be attached to the legs, since limb move-ments can also disturb sleep. Men suffering from impotence may also have sensors attached to other regions, although this has become less necessary since the advent of Viagra (see page 20).

must know
Sleep disorder help
Most sleep disorders centres investigate sleep-related respiratory disorders. Parasomnias (see page 143) may be investigated. Insomnias are rarely investigated, partly because of the three main outcomes of a recording:
1. The insomniac sleeps all night – for the first time in a while
2. The insomniac does not sleep at all – or that is their complaint.
3. The objective recording does not match the subjective complaint – which can create a problem.

What happens next

The wires all connect up to a junction box somewhere near the head of the bed, so it is possible for you to turn around on the bed. Technicians will then go through a routine of testing the connections, by getting you to move your eyes to the right and left, closing them, stopping and starting breathing, and so on. It's then a simple matter of falling asleep and letting the EEG do its work. Brain activity readings are reproduced on the computer screen in the form of a hypnogram or polysomnograph while you sleep (see page 185). Some centres will also prefer to video you during the night as this can be helpful in interpreting some of the electrophysiological data. The whole measurement procedure is called polysomnography and is the major diagnostic tool in sleep disorders, particularly in the evaluation of suspected sleep-related breathing disorders and Periodic Limb Movement Disorder (PLMD – see page 150), when the cause of insomnia is uncertain and when behavioural or pharmacological therapies have been unsuccessful. Many sleep disorders do not require polysomnography for diagnosis but it can invaluable when it has been impossible to obtain a definitive diagnosis using other measures.

Patients often worry about not being able to sleep in the laboratory, but the majority, particularly if their problem is excessive sleepiness, do so. Conditioned insomniacs may also, embarrassingly, sleep well. This should not be a problem as most centres will be aware of both the pitfalls and the benefits of the measurement techniques used.

must know

Tests

These include overnight recordings, daytime sleep (patients are told to sleep) and wakefulness tests (patients are told to remain awake while they are lying down in a dark, comfortable room). Some people may be asked to perform a task, such as a simple simulation of car driving. For Restless Leg Syndrome (see page 151) there is SIT (the Suggested Immobilization Test) which is increasingly being used. In this test patients are told to sit or lie down with legs outstretched. The legs have sensors attached which measure leg movement and the patients are asked every five minutes how uncomfortable their legs feel.

Sleep medicine accreditation

The American Sleep Disorders Association (ASDA) provides an accreditation service for sleep disorder centres and laboratories. ASDA's standards are updated annually and the association ensures that facilities maintain the highest quality of patient care. Re-accreditation is required every five years. Sleep medicine specialists in the US are accredited by the American Board of Sleep Medicine and may be either medical doctors or have PhDs in a sleep-related speciality. There is no equivalent in the UK as the methods of analyzing sleep are considered too complex. The technologists who do this work are accredited by the US Board of Registered Poly-somnographic Technicians, who have the initials RPSGT after their names. The RPSGT accreditation is now also being increasingly accepted in the UK.

Other tests

Apart from polysomnography, other tests include the Sleep Latency test (which measures how long it takes you to fall asleep). Variations of this are also used, such as the Multiple Sleep Latency test (in which 4–6 measurements are repeatedly taken after a series of naps following a night's rest), to measure daytime sleepiness; and the Multiple Wakefulness test, used to measure your ability to stay awake.

Treatments for sleep disorders

There are many methods of treating sleep problems, from herbal remedies to light therapy. The ones most likely to be recommended by specialist sleep centres and doctors are given below. Used singly or in combination, they can provide effective solutions to many major sleep disorders.

Cognitive Behavioural Therapy (CBT)

This is becoming an increasingly popular method of treating chronic insomnias such as psychophysiological insomnia (see page 129). All cognitive behaviour therapies work on the basis of changing behaviour by replacing negative thoughts with positive ones. The idea is that most 'unhealthy' patterns of thinking have been learned over a period of time – and can be 'unlearned' with specialist strategies. All CBT therapists are trained psychologists, but sleep CBT therapists take normal CBT one step further because of the specialist knowledge of sleep behaviour that is required. In general, sleep CBT will involve giving the patient information on sleep, suggesting behavioural modifications and dealing with thoughts that might adversely impact on sleep onset. Typical examples are shown below:

Sleep information
- nature and function of sleep
- sleep needs
- general health and lifestyle
- environmental influences

Sleep behaviour
Including pre-sleep behaviour and scheduling (like those described in the diary section of pages 98–101)
- sleep restriction procedures

- stimulus control
- relaxation techniques (e.g. progressive relaxation)
- mind control techniques (e.g. worry management, controlling a racing mind, reducing sleep effort)

General cognitive therapy
- managing anxiety and intrusive thoughts
- challenging maladaptive thoughts (self-worth, value of sleep)

Common behavioural techniques
Here are two typical exercises a CBT practitioner might suggest:
- Set aside about 30 minutes a day exclusively for worrying! This will help stop you worrying all the time and will at least begin to restrict it. During the worry period, keep a journal on the type of worries you have. The very act of writing them down may help to reduce them.
- Before going to bed, sit down and take a few minutes to anticipate the worries you might have in bed. Write them down. Don't spend time thinking about them, because you might not be able to stop! Just set them aside. Another way is to sit with your eyes closed, imagine the worry as if it was a balloon floating in the air, and mentally burst it. This should take only 5–10 minutes, and when you have finished you may want to spend a few moments enjoying your uncluttered mind.

must know
CBT
Findings from controlled clinical trials indicate that 70–80 per cent of insomniacs benefit from CBT.

Insomniacs should never 'try to sleep' – that effort is often counterproductive. CBT therapists will instruct insomniacs on how to let go of wakefulness instead of trying to sleep. Also, an insomniac may become very aware of what their body and mind are doing prior to going to sleep and at sleep onset, so distraction techniques are taught to draw attention away from the natural process of going to sleep. Finally, insomniacs can develop many negative thoughts about themselves and their ability to do anything. For instance, if they look at the clock and find that it is very late, their thinking can run along several negative paths: 'I can't even fall asleep' – 'I can't do anything right' – 'I'm not asleep yet, how am I going to manage tomorrow?' – 'I've lost control of my life.' The negative thinking can be emotional, resulting in anxiety, irritation and despair, none of which is conducive to sleep. CBT helps bring this thinking out into the open so that it can be dealt with head on during the day, enabling emotional response to be weakened or countered during the night.

Stimulants in the treatment of narcolepsy and other hypersomnia conditions

Narcolepsy (see page 137) not only consists of problems with apparently spontaneous and irresistible sleep; it also includes muscle paralysis and poor nocturnal sleep. Medicinal treatments often aim to tackle each aspect. Amphetamines and methylphenidate were used in the past as stimulants but they have been replaced by modafinil. This does not control the cataplexy (see page 184) and so tricyclic antidepressants are used for this. More recently gammahydroxybutyrate, in the form of sodium oxybate, has emerged (though not yet licensed in many countries) as a treatment that controls both sleepiness and cataplexy. In addition, the night-time symptoms are sometimes controlled using hypnotics.

Medical treatments for RLS

In addition to the experience of discomfort in their legs, Restless Leg Syndrome (see pages 151) sufferers have a biological clock that prevents them from falling asleep in the evening. Treatment of RLS may include conservative measures (see page 170) as well as prescribed medications in severe cases. Treatment often requires medicines that are similar to those used in Parkinson's Disease (see page 162), such as L-Dopa, although this is too powerful a compound to be used routinely. In recent years, two new compounds have been developed: pramipexole or ropinirole. Sometimes patients can not take L-Dopa type medicines, in which case there are alternatives although they are not as efficacious (e.g. oxycodone or dihydrocodeine).

Sleeping pills

For many people, sleeping pills are the first port of call when they have a bout of insomnia, and billions are spent on sleeping prescriptions every year. But while sleeping potions and pills have been used for generations, they have invariably caused unwanted side-effects, and classes of drug that were regarded as an advance in one generation have fallen out of favour in the next. Barbiturates were once seen as excellent sleeping pills, but the often fatal effects of overdosing (as in the case of Ernest Hemingway and possibly of Marilyn Monroe) led to them being replaced by benzodiazepines. These were found to be generally safe on overdose, but problems with tolerance (getting used to the drug so that higher doses are needed to achieve the same effect) or dependence (not being able to get off the pill) or rebound (problems with exacerbation of symptoms upon withdrawal) have now cast a pall over these compounds.

must know

Sleeping pills
Most sleeping pills have been developed to be taken at a conventional bedtime. They shouldn't be used in the middle of the night.

More recently, a class of pills called 'z' pills, so-called because of the zs in some of their generic names (zolpidem, zaleplon, zopiclone, etc.), has been introduced, which acts on receptors in a similar way to benzodiazepines in promoting sleep. However, after looking across a number of studies totalling 3909 patients, the UK's National Institute of Clinical Excellence (NICE) found that there were few clear, consistent differences between these and the benzodiazepines. Their conclusion was that, overall, prescription of benzodiazepines was still warranted.

In practice, general practitioners are reticent to prescribe sleeping pills, mainly because of NHS recommendation to limit prescribing to short courses. They often use low doses of the older antidepressants dothiepin and amitriptyline because of their sedative properties. There is also a good argument for using

Commonly used sleeping pills

Benzodiazepines

temazepam
nitrazepam
lormetazepam
diazepam

'z' drugs

zolpidem
zopiclone
zaleplon

Also used by specialists

clonazepam (benzodiazepine)
venlafaxine (antidepressant akin to SSRIs)
mirtazapine (antidepressant akin to SSRIs)
trazodone (antidepressant akin to TCA)

Also used by GPs

Antidepressants
dothiepin (TCA)
amitriptyline (TCA)

Over the counter

diphenhydramine (antihistamine)

antidepressants as there is a strong association between insomnia and depression. Over-the-counter compounds of products such as diphenhydramine can be bought at the chemist's (Dipenhydramine was originally developed as an antihistamine, but its side-effect of daytime drowsiness was so noticeable it was redeveloped as a sleeping aid!)

Pros	Cons
Will help to promote sleep in most cases	Possibility of dependence (unable to sleep without taking sleeping pills) Tolerance (pills stopping working over time) Falling Hangover effects Road traffic accidents
Will help to promote sleep in most cases	Fewer side-effects than the benzodiazepines, but more expensive
Clonazepam – same as the benzodiazepines Antidepressant, may help to wind down the brain (not the typical anti-depression effect). Some are soporfic	Clonazepam – same as the benzodiazepines; not licensed for sleeping pill usage
Antidepressant, may help to wind down the brain (not the typical anti-depression effect). TCAs are soporific	Limited evidence of effects on sleep
Will help to aid sleep onset. Less effective than prescribed sleeping pills	Effects on sleep decline rapidly Morning grogginess and hangover if taken too late at night Not as efficacious as benzodiazepines or 'z' drugs

Light therapy

Light therapy, in which patients are exposed to bright lights for extended periods, has been found to be especially useful in treating circadian rhythm disorders such as Advanced Sleep Phase Syndrome and Delayed Sleep Phase Syndrome (see pages 140–41), and Seasonal Affective Disorder (SAD – see page 17). The internal bodyclock is affected by light that passes to the brain via the retina. If this connection is somehow affected, it can disrupt the body's natural circadian rhythm. Exposing the affected individuals to bright lights during the day can often make the body clock keep 'correct' time. Light therapy is administered using light boxes that produce between 2500 and 10,000 lux (lux being the measurement of light density). The length of daily exposure will vary according to the strength of light applied, but will usually involve daily sessions ranging from 20 minutes to two hours. You may have to adjust your routine to find what works best. See also Chapter 1 and Melatonin (page 16) .

must know

Shift workers

Light therapy is frequently used to help shift workers adjust to their schedules. The first people to use light therapy in this way was NASA, the US space agency.

Melatonin supplements

Studies have established that low-level melatonin supplementation may promote sleep in some (but not all) poor sleepers if given at different times during the day. It will not, however, change nocturnal sleep in normal sleepers. Rather than affecting sleep itself, melatonin (see page 16) is believed to be a gentle physiological modulator of the sleep process that leads to a state resembling 'quiet wakefulness'. Effects vary from person to person, and because melatonin is produced in the gut as well as the brain, its impact may be increased after the intake of other nutritional substances such as tryptophan (see page 77). Melatonin has proved to be successful in the treatment of Seasonal Affective Disorder (SAD – see also page 17).

Melatonin legislation

Melatonin was initially regarded as a nutritional supplement and a safe natural product but in the mid-1990s, following international publicity on its purported benefits in some countries, it switched in status from a nutritional supplement to a medicine. For most natural product manufacturers, the expense of acquiring medical licensing in such a case means, ironically, that their products are withdrawn from the market. And this is what happened with melatonin. In 1995, the UK's Medicines Control Agency (MCA), deciding that melatonin was 'medicinal by function' and therefore required a licence, ordered suppliers to stop selling melatonin supplements until they had obtained the licence. Similarly, in 1996 Germany's Federal Institute for Drugs and Medical Devices also decided that melatonin's use had become medicinal and therefore needed medicinal marketing authorization, a decision that was shared by Norway. In 1997, New Zealand re-classified melatonin as a prescription medicine saying the information on its safety and efficacy was insufficient – considerations that had not been significant when it had been unclassified.

must know

Supplements
Melatonin secretion from the pineal gland reduces with age, so supplementation seems reasonable. Iron supplementation is also used in sleep medicine as it helps prevent the development of Restless Leg Syndrome and fatigue and tiredness. More recently it has been found that the concentration of creatine goes down in the brain after sleep deprivation and that supplementation can partly counteract this. Supplements are best taken under supervision as it is possible to overdose on some varieties.

Chronotherapy

Chronotherapy is a form of treatment in which clocks are used to adjust misalignments of the internal bodyclock by moving bed-times and rising times until normal sleep/awake is achieved. It is used for circadian rhythm sleep disorders (see page 139) and has been found to be particularly useful in treating Delayed Sleep Phase Syndrome (DSPS – see page 141), in which people go to bed and wake up increasingly late. In such cases, the aim of chronotherapy will be to move bed and rising times later each day until normal times are achieved. The table opposite shows how it might work over two week courses of treatment, in which the DSPS sufferer goes to bed three hours later each day until their bodyclock is correctly aligned.

As part of the rescheduling involves sleeping during the day, it may be necessary to use this kind of programme over a holiday period or make special arrangement with your employer. An advantage of this programme is that it is drug-free, but the dis-advantage is that it takes a long time to run, and the new bed and rise times have to be strictly followed as there is a danger of slippage. Once the new time is established, it may also be necessary to use bright light and exercise programmes to keep the internal clock running to the conventional time. The alter-natives to this are still experimental but may include the use of melatonin.

Chronotherapy as described here for the control of DSPS is but one approach. Using daylight, exercise, eating and social interaction as synchronizing cues can also help. Other forms of chronotherapy are applied to disruptions to sleep associated with other disorders,

Typical chronotherapy programme

Day 1:	sleep 3 a.m. to 11 a.m.
Day 2:	sleep 4 a.m. to noon
Day 3:	sleep 5 a.m. to 1 p.m.
Day 4:	sleep 6 a.m. to 2 p.m.
Day 5:	sleep 7 a.m. to 3 p.m.
Day 6:	sleep 8 a.m. to 4 p.m.
Day 7:	sleep 9 a.m. to 5 p.m.
Day 8:	sleep 10 a.m. to 6 p.m.
Day 9:	sleep 11 a.m. to 7 p.m.
Day 10:	sleep noon to 8 p.m.
Day 11:	sleep 1 p.m. to 9 p.m.
Day 12:	sleep 2 p.m. to 10 p.m.
Day 13:	sleep 3 p.m. to 11 p.m
Day 14:	sleep 4 p.m. to midnight
Day 15:	sleep 5 p.m. to 1 a.m.
Day 16:	sleep 6 p.m. to 2 a.m.
Day 17:	sleep 7 p.m. to 3 a.m.
Day 18:	sleep 8 p.m. to 4 a.m.
Day 19:	sleep 9 p.m. to 5 a.m.
Day 20:	sleep 10 p.m. to 6 a.m.
Day 21:	sleep 11 p.m. to 7 a.m.

such asthma attacks at night or the blood pressure surge and related heart attacks and strokes in the morning. Treatments are timed to be most effective according to the particular disorder. Consequently, chronotherapy should be carried out under strict medical supervision, as it may interfere with prescribed medicines (chronotherapeutics). Many doctors will be aware of chronotherapy although they may not be sure of the details as this is a new therapeutic approach. Referral to a specialist is advisable.

Common CPAP problems and solutions

The mask feels uncomfortable. try different masks until you find one that fits well.

Dry and stuffy nose. try using a humidifier to moisten the air from the CPAP device.

Blocked-up nose. ask your doctor whether a nasal spray might help.

The mask irritates your skin and nose. Try different masks, or skin moisturizers especially made for CPAP users. (Some petroleum-based products can damage the mask, so check what's suitable.) Nasal pillows that relieve pressure on the bridge of the nose may help. Try alternating between a regular CPAP mask one night and nasal pillows the next.

The mask leaks air. Some people can't keep their jaw closed while wearing the mask. A chin strap can help hold up your jaw to keep the air in.

The pressure is annoying. Find out if there are more appropriate machines that control the pressure differently.

The mask slips off during sleep or you don't wear it every night. Most people can't wear the mask all night long, every night, right from the start. Keep trying, even if you can only use the mask for an hour a night at first. It all helps and you will get used to it.

Continuous Positive Airway Pressure (CPAP)

The CPAP device is a common form of treatment for sleep-related breathing disorders and especially Obstructive Sleep Apnoea (OSA – see page 132).

A typical CPAP device consists of a mask attached to a tube and a type of fan that blows pressurized air into the mask. The air pressure keeps the airway open so that air can pass through the throat into the lungs.

CPAP devices may not cure OSA, but they will alleviate the symptoms and prevent the development of associated health problems such as high blood pressure. Some people take to them straight away, with dramatic improvements in daytime alertness and feelings of wellbeing, but many can have problems with them, especially at first. Talking to other users, or support groups, may be helpful.

CPAP nasal mask

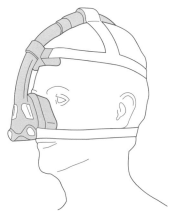

want to know more?

Other sources
- A good source of general information on OSA and most topics is www.nhsdirect.com
- For information about pills in general, see the NHS National Prescribing Centre. www.npc.co.uk
- For more controversial views on sleeping pills, see www.benzo.org.uk. See also Dan Kripke, The Dark Side of Sleeping Pills
- For information about anxiety and depression, see: www.livinglifetothefull.com, www.dascot.org (Depression Alliance), www.moodgym.anu.edu.au (the MoodGYM – online prevention of depression) and www.beyondblue.org.au (Australian national depression initiative)

Glossary

Actigraph
Electronic device used to measure the brain and thus wakefulness and sleep. It usually takes the form of a wristwatch.

Advanced Sleep Phase Syndrome (ASPS)
Also called Phase Advance. Bodyclock disorder causing a chronic inability to stay awake in the evening and/or sleep later in the morning. It is one of the two main types of *circadian rhythm disorder*. See also *Delayed Sleep Phase Syndrome (DSPS)*.

Alpha
Brain waves of a frequency of 8–12 cycles/second are called alpha waves. They are most often seen in relaxed wakefulness with closed eyes. However, they may also be seen in combination with delta waves in conditions such as fibromyalgia.

Anchor sleep
Fixed period of about four hours slept every day while on a shift rotation.

Autogenics
Relaxation technique involving a series of attention-focusing exercises specifically designed to induce relaxation.

Cataplexy
Muscular weakness ranging from a slight slackening of the facial muscles to total collapse. It is frequently found in people with narcolepsy.

Chronotherapeutics
Medical prescription which not only dictates the dose but also the precise time at which the medicine should be taken (to take account of circadian rhythms and sleep).

Chronotherapy
Form of treatment in which clocks are used to adjust misalignments of the bodyclock. It is useful in *circadian rhythm disorders*.

Circadian rhythm disorders
Disorders of the internal body clock. The two most common types are *Advanced Sleep Phase Syndrome (ASPS)* and *Delayed Phase Syndrome (DSPS)*.

Cognitive Behavioural Therapy (CBT)
Form of therapy that seeks to identify and challenge negative thought processes as well as directly dealing with behaviour that is not conducive to sleep. It is commonly used in treating sleep disorders.

Continuous Positive Airway Pressure (CPAP) device
Device used to keep the airways open so that air can pass through the throat into the lungs.

Delayed Sleep Phase Syndrome (DSPS)
Also called Phase Delay. Bodyclock disorder causing progressively later and later bedtimes. It is one of the two main types of *circadian rhythm disorder*. See also *Advanced Sleep Phase Syndrome (ASPS)*.

Delta sleep
Alternative term for slow-wave sleep.

Electro-encephalogram (EEG)
Machine used to record the electrical activity of the brain, or brainwaves.

Electromyogram (EMG)
Machine used to measure muscle movements during sleep.

Electro-oculogram (EOG)
Machine used to record eye movements during sleep.

Epworth Sleepiness Scale (ESS)
Scale used to rate sleepiness during daytime activities.

Hyperarousal
State of increased activity in the brain and body. It is characterized by an increase in heart rate, breathing and sweating.

Hypersomnias
Group of sleep disorders characterized by excessive day-time sleep. The most common type of hypersomnia is *narcolepsy*.

Hypertension
Medical term for high blood pressure.

Hypnogram
Recording of sleep activity in the brain. See also *Polysomnograph*.

Hypothalamus
Small cone-shaped structure in the brain that regulates many functions of the body, including sleep.

Hypoxia
Lack of oxygen in the tissues.

Insomnia
Umbrella term used to describe a general inability to fall asleep or stay asleep. There are many types. It can be transient (lasting only a few days), short-term (lasting a few weeks) or chronic (lasting for months or years).

Light therapy
Treatment involving exposure to bright lights. It is frequently used to treat *Seasonal Affective Disorder (SAD)*.

Lux
Measurement of the density of light.

Melatonin
Hormone secreted by the pineal gland in the brain. It tells the brain when it is dark. Also available (in some countries) in the form of supplements.

Multiple Sleep Latency Test
Test used to measure daytime sleepiness. It involves a series of naps taken after a full night's sleep.

Obstructive Sleep Apnoea (OSA)
The most common of all breathing-related sleep disorders, caused by narrowing of the upper airway during sleep.

Oximetry
Method of measuring oxygen in the blood. It usually involves attaching a probe to a finger.

Parasomnias
Group of sleeping disorders involving either movement during sleep or seeing, hearing or feeling things that are not real. The most common form is sleepwalking.

Glossary

Polysomnograph/polysomnogram
Alternative term for *Hypnogram*.

Rapid Eye Movement sleep
REM. The last, and deepest, stage of sleep, in which dreaming occurs.

Seasonal Affective Disorder (SAD)
Type of depression in which sufferers find it impossible to get up on dark winter mornings. It is believed to be caused by a lack of *melatonin*.

Serotonin
A chemical produced in the brain that is associated with sleep and general well-being.

Sleep Bruxism
Medical term for tooth grinding at night.

Sleep debt
Term for progressive lack of sleep that needs to be recovered.

Sleep enuresis
Medical term for bedwetting.

Sleep hygiene
Term used to describe lifestyle, environmental and general health issues that can affect sleep.

Sleep Latency test
Test used to assess the length of time between going to bed and the onset of sleep.

Slow-wave sleep
Term used to describe Stages 3 and 4 of sleep. See also *Delta sleep*.

Sonambulism
Medical term for sleepwalking.

Suprachiasmatic Nucleus (SCN)
The brain's biological clock. It helps to synchronize sleep with the body's natural circadian rhythm.

Tryptophan
Essential amino acid available in the diet that is believed to improve sleep.

Uvulopalatopharyngoplasty (UVPP)
Surgical procedure of opening the airways. It is used to treat snoring.

Useful addresses

British Sleep Society (BSS)
PO Box 247
Colne
Huntingdon
PE28 3UZ
The British Sleep Society is a professional organization, a registered charity for medical, scientific and healthcare workers dealing with sleeping disorders. It does not deal directly with the public.

British Snoring & Sleep Apnoea Association
Castle Court
41 London Road
Reigate
Surrey
RH2 9RJ
Support organization.
Tel (helpline): 0800 085 1097
Tel (administration): 01737 245638
Web: www.britishsnoring.co.uk
Telephone: Mon–Fri, 9 a.m. to 5 p.m.

CRY-SIS Helpline
BM CRY-SIS
London
WC1N 3XX
Support for parents
Tel: 08451 228 669
Telephone: 365 days a year, 9 a.m. to 10 p.m.
Web: www.cry-sis.org.uk

Ekbom Support Group
18 Rodbridge Drive
Thorpe Bay
Essex
SS1 3DF
Tel: 01702 582002
Web: www.ekbom.org.uk
Patient support group
Telephone: Mon/Wed/Fri from 10 a.m. to 2 p.m. Other times on answerphone

Narcolepsy Association (UK)
UKAN
50 Culver Street
Newent
Gloucestershire
GL18 1DA
Patient support group
Web: www.narcolepsy.org.uk
Tel: 0845 4500 394 (answering machine at all times)

Scottish Association for Sleep Apnoea
The Kestrels
54 Abbotsford Road
Galashiels
Selkirkshire
TD1 3HP
Tel: 01896 758675
Telephone: any evening except Mon/Wed/Thurs

Sleep Apnoea Trust
12a Bakers Piece
Kingston Blount
Oxon
OX39 4SW
Patient support group
Tel: 0845 60 60 685 (answering machine available)
Fax: 0845 60 60 685
Web: www.sleep-apnoea-trust.org

Sleep Council
High Corn Mill
Chapel Hill
Skipton
North Yorkshire
BD23 1NL
The Sleep Council is a non-profit organization, limited by guarantee and funded by bed manufacturers, retailers and suppliers and has funded an insomnia telephone support number for many years. Its aim is to advise and reassure those who are having trouble sleeping.
Tel (for leaflet requests): 0800 0187 923 (24-hour answerphone)
Tel (office): 01756 791089
Fax: 01756 798789
Web: www.sleepcouncil.com
Email: info@sleepcouncil.org.uk
Telephone (helpline): 020 8994 9874, Mon–Fri, 6–8 p.m.

Sleep Scotland
8 Hope Park Square
Edinburgh
EH8 9NW
Scotland
A service dedicated to helping the families of children with special needs and severe sleep problems by training and supporting sleep counsellors throughout Scotland.
Telephone: 0131 651 1392
Fax: 0131 651 1392

Index

Index